KILL THE DEMON?

WM Publications
Elandsgracht 35
1016 TN Amsterdam

Original title : Tuer le Démon?
English translation by Armèle Desmarchelier

Front cover illustration. "Mount Cameroon Demon" by Sebastian Rypson
Back cover photo Pete Purnell
All inside photos Paul Schäublin unless otherwise mentioned
Map page 7 design Leszek Sczaniecki

A NOTE TO THE READER:
This is an autobiographical story without any scientific pretension. All medical references included in this book are the result of author's own research and are based on his own interpretation.
 All matters regarding your health and wellbeing require medical supervision. Neither the author nor publisher shall be liable or responsible for any loss, injury, or damage allegedly arising from information or suggestion in this book.

All profit on the sales of this book will be donated to the Prinses Beatrix Spierfonds (Princess Beatrice Muscle Fund) which carries out studies in the field of muscle diseases. See <www.prinsesbeatrixspierfonds.nl>

ISBN: 978-90-830040-0-6

First Edition, June 2019

KILL THE DEMON?

MY GUILLAIN-BARRÉ EXPERIENCE

PAUL SCHÄUBLIN

WM PUBLICATIONS
2019

CONTENT

Chad
N'Djamena
Nigeria
Lagos
Cameroon
Mount Cameroon
Douala
Luanda
Angola

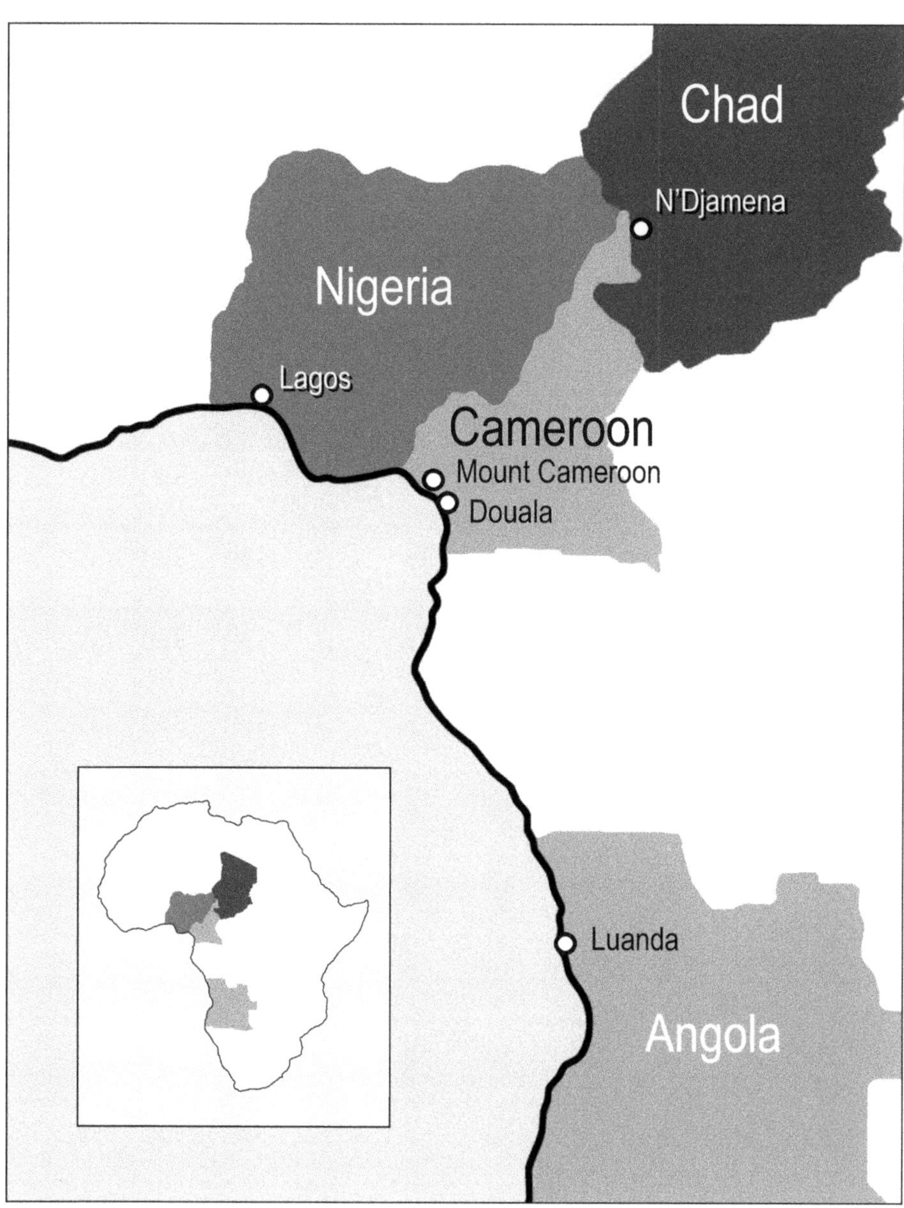

Africa

INTRODUCTION

This story is about my experience with this rare disorder called Guillain-Barré syndrome (GBS), which affected me back in 2006 and significantly impacted the rest of my life. A story of hope with a positive outcome.

I originally wrote this account for myself – to some extent as a therapeutic exercise – and to share with family and friends. I later decided to proceed with publication in order to share with all those interested and especially those affected by a similar disease.

Some say it is a story of courage. That's not how I would describe it, since I didn't really have a choice. For me it was just a normal way of doing, guided by patience and a sort of natural optimism it seems I have embedded in me.

To those affected by this mysterious disease: be patient, never give up, fight, you will get better.

Please note this is a narrative essay without any scientific pretension. All medical references included herein are the result of my own research and are based on my own interpretation.

Some of the photos included are made with my phone. Apologies for the poor quality, I still thought it was still worth including them as a matter of information.

Perhaps all the dragons in our lives are princesses who are only waiting to see us act, with beauty and courage.

Perhaps everything that frightens us is, in its deepest essence, something helpless that wants our love.

– Rainer Maria Rilke

CHAPTER ONE

LAGOS

Lagos Airport, Tuesday November 28, 2006. The ambulance taking me to my emergency evacuation has been held up in front of the gate to the tarmac. The engine is ticking over.

Outside, I can hear my doctor and the ambulance driver arguing with the security guards. They are speaking in dialect and I can't understand a word. The discussion becomes heated, they are having a row.

I am lying in the ambulance unable to move. I am not in pain; I am paralysed.

The palaver drags on, they are yelling and arguing furiously. The doctor opens the door and explains that the document to give us direct access to the tarmac needs an official stamp. The heat from outside rushes into the vehicle. It's moist, humid and unpleasant. He closes down the door and the air-conditioning coolness regains the upper hand. Thank goodness there is airco.

I have my mobile with me and as luck would have it there is a network. I call my wife Wanda who is in Europe and doesn't know about my situation yet:

"I am paralysed, I cannot move but I'm not in any pain. It started yesterday. I am now in an ambulance at Lagos airport, and they are going to evacuate me to Geneva in a special plane. Do not worry too much, they say it is for the best and that I will be better taken care of in Europe".

I can imagine how worried she must be. By coincidence, she happens to be in Geneva, just about to board a plane back to Amsterdam, where we live.

"Shall I stay in Geneva?"

"No, you'd better go back home. You have no place to stay, it will take time before we arrive in Geneva. They said I will get better. Don't worry. I will call you as soon as I arrive. Go home, you will be able to see me when things have cleared up a bit. The flight from Geneva to Amsterdam is only one hour".

Wanda had just spent a few days in our small chalet in the Swiss Alps with her friend Magda. They had already checked in and are about to board. I manage to convince them and they catch their flight.

If Wanda had seen the state I was in she would probably have stayed in Geneva. But she could have done nothing to help and would have been even more worried. It was better this way.

After about twenty minutes, the shouting finally stops. I do not know exactly how the problem was solved and no one tells me. A superior has probably been called in. Everything is negotiable in this country. A missing stamp on a document is disastrous as it's a welcome source of income, especially when a foreigner is involved. In general, the only way to manage is to baksheesh. The endless arguing is probably because my companions are refusing to pay. The doctor returns and sits next to me without saying a word, still visibly annoyed. The ambulance moves, drives through the gate and heads towards the aircraft. But after only a few metres, we stop again. The rear door of the ambulance opens and a man in overalls asks for my passport so that he can process the custom formalities.

The doctor asks in an aggressive tone: "Who are you, do you work for the customs department?"

He replies: "No."

"Then I won't give you the passport. I will wait until a customs officer comes."

The other man doesn't insist, closes the door and the ambulance resumes its sluggish pace. The doctor understands the 'official' only too well. Swiss passports are a desirable commodity in this part of the world, they can easily reach 1,000 francs on the black market.

We hear our plane is not here yet and we have to wait. In the meantime, an official customs employee, at least I hope so, has taken my passport to his office to have it stamped. So we wait. Luckily the ambulance has airco. It must be around 10 am.

THE MEGALOPOLIS

I had arrived in Lagos a few days earlier, on Thursday 23 November, after a week's holiday at my home in Amsterdam.

I'm a civil engineer, who worked for an oil company (ExxonMobil). As project manager, I was responsible for the renovation of the administrative headquarters of our Nigerian branch. This huge 8 storey building was built in the early 1990s and housed about a thousand employees and auxiliaries.

This was my third visit to Nigeria for this new project, which I recently joined. I was managing it in addition to two other office construction projects, one in N'Djamena in Chad and the other in Douala in Cameroon. Both projects were now well underway and required less supervision from me.

Lagos was a gigantic megacity with an unknown number of inhabitants. 15 million, 20 million? Those were the figures put forward at the time, but nobody knew exactly how many people lived here. It was a huge human anthill, built on and around a lagoon, the ultimate concrete 'jungle'.

As I left Lagos airport, I was confronted with a sea of people standing behind the security barriers. I had to spot a man in red overalls who was supposed to welcome me and take me to the bus chartered by the company to take me to my hotel. No easy task, especially in the muggy, suffocating heat.

Each time I arrived here, I was overcome by the same anxiety. Will the man in red be there as agreed? What will I do if he isn't? Who should I turn to without running the risk of being swindled (a real risk that other visitors have fallen victim to)?

This was one of the reasons why people waiting for visitors were no longer authorized to wait inside the airport with a little sign bearing the traveller's name. In the past, thugs had managed to obtain lists of the names of travellers and would then wait for them with false signs. Unsuspecting visitors would be driven somewhere isolated, robbed and abandoned to their fate. Although this practice was not really commonplace, it was still a risk.

So the company had opted for an employee in red overalls (red being the company's colour). And to my great relief, there he was in the corner, 50 metres to the right, as planned.

Five other passengers arrived, all expats working for the company. Probably they had shared my anxieties at the terminal exit. We had all arrived on the Air France flight from Paris. Although we thought we were complete, the small bus chartered by the company did not move. The others seemed rather depressed and did not speak much. They had the expat's blues: that sinking feeling when you returned to work after your annual or bi-annual leave. With a heavy heart you started counting the days until your next holiday. That was not my situation, as I had only worked abroad for relatively short periods, with visitor status. The driver had been ordered to wait for the British Airways flight from London, which was carrying other company employees. I heard the others moan. This meant an hour's wait, fortunately with the engine running in order to operate the air conditioning. The windows were covered with white curtains to prevent anyone from looking inside and getting any funny ideas. It was past 6 pm and night had fallen.

The other passengers finally arrived and the bus started, much to our relief. Nobody talked, everyone was eager to arrive safely, have a shower and rest after their long and often gruelling journey. Most of us had travelled from Houston, Texas, via Paris or London. We were escorted by two police cars, one in front and one behind us, the flashing lights on their roof emitting blinding blue flashes.

On my first visit to Nigeria a few years earlier, I was very impressed by this. Now I was used to it. I noticed that many vehicles in the traffic also had spinning lights on the roof. Either there were a lot of official cars or they were really easy to acquire on the black market. I inclined towards the second explanation. These lights were supposed to help the vehicle make its way through the heavy traffic, but so many cars had them that they were no help at all. Lagos's traffic was incredibly dense at any time of the day with everyone tooting their horn, as if that could speed things up.

The 'Expressway' connected the airport to the city and crossed the entire city, which was built on islands, with a long bridge stretching across the lagoon. At rush hour, the traffic soon got congested. Whenever possible, cars went through the verge to overtake other vehicles. There were no rules, everything goes and as a result, the traffic jams were incredible. Everyone was hooting, the revolving lights turned and flashed and the sirens shred our eardrums. Suddenly, everything ground to a halt. A bus stop on the side of the motorway had caused a massive holdup. Minibuses double-parked to pick up passengers would only leave when they were full. This created a funnel effect. The vehicles drove fast, trying to overtake, squeezed up, brushed against each other, got stuck or got to the shoulder of the road. Inspectors on the crowded minibuses perched on the lowest step, clinging to the door frame that has been left open, almost getting crushed by the next vehicle. One inspector missed being hit by just a few millimetres, but he did not even flinch, as if this was a perfectly normal occurrence. Soon there were three, four, maybe five queues slowly rolling side-by-side and all of a sudden the road was transformed into a huge market. Vendors passed between cars, selling absolutely everything: water, 'fresh' drinks, sweets, cookies, steering wheel trims, newspapers, car mats, toilet paper, toys, fruits, etc. They came one after the other, risking their lives between the cars, clutching each other. This went on for at least 200 metres if not more.

But this time, there was relatively little traffic. We were at the end of the day and driving against the current, towards the city. We managed to cover 30 kilometres in 40 minutes. We left the bridge and stopped at a red light: one of the few traffic lights I had ever seen in Nigeria. I drew back the curtain and discovered the hallucinatory spectacle of a small city of people living under the Expressway bridge, cooking and making fires for light, housed in improvised shelters, some taking advantage of the traffic lights to beg from stopped vehicles. There was no noise, everything was quiet; some people were busy cooking, others bargaining with each other, yet others were just sitting and watching as the children played. The traffic light turned green and the bus turned onto the Lekki Expressway and 10 minutes later we arrived at our hotel.

We were on Victoria Island, one of the "safest" residential and business areas of the city where many of the international companies were located. That was where my company had its headquarters: Mobil House.

The Lekki Expressway, a dual carriageway, passed by the foot of the hotel. By day, the traffic was very dense. Everyone was in a hurry, it was one big horn concert from dawn to dusk. The hotel, rented by the company and only inhabited by employees and consultants, was about 200 metres from the headquarters on the other side of the road. Anyone who tried to cross on foot at that time of day was suicidal. As we were strongly advised against going on foot, minibuses took us from the hotel to Mobil House. But after 8 pm everything suddenly became quiet. People did not drive at night.

THE MOBIL HOUSE RENOVATION PROJECT

This was my third visit to this project. I replaced a Canadian colleague, Bob Weir, who had just retired. It was a huge renovation project which involved replacing all the furniture and floors, updating air conditioning and computers, modernizing elevators and completely transforming the kitchens and canteen. Technically, it was a relatively simple operation but extremely complex from the organizational point of view, due to the fact that the building was occupied. The works had been planned in phases, spread over a period of at least two years.

We were at the end of the preparatory phase, the budget had been approved and the specifications were ready. The tender for construction companies was about to be issued and talks with pre-qualified companies were scheduled for the coming week.

The project team I supervised comprised four people:

Samuel Nbuisi, a Nigerian I met in Chad, where he came for an internship, he was in charge of Security;

Nkechi Onaijde, a Nigerian delegate of the Human Resources department, she was responsible for internal communication linked to the progress of the works;

Nigel Manning, a South African consultant in charge of design and construction follow-up;

Andy Buttery, a British consultant in charge of planning and organizing the internal migrations (relocations) of the various departments: 1,000 people to be "migrated" from one place to another inside the building, in different phases, over a period of about two years. Not exactly a walk in the park.

THE CHAD-CAMEROON PROJECT

One month earlier, in early November 2006, before my leave in Amsterdam, I had spent two weeks in Douala, Cameroon, for one of the two other projects I was responsible for: the construction of the headquarters of COTCO, the Cameroon Oil Transport Company, a subsidiary of ExxonMobil. It was a small three-storey building housing 150 employees. The construction started in spring 2006 and was scheduled to last two years.

A small project team of five people were responsible for monitoring the work. A 100% Cameroonian team, which managed the project well, worked under the direction of my colleague and friend Jean-Michel Tolen, director of works.

I was very involved in the preparations for this project and was responsible for the design, the budget, selecting companies and, of course, liaising with the client. Now all I had to do was conduct monthly supervision visits.

This construction was part of the Chad–Cameroon oil exploitation project. The oil fields were located in southern Chad and a 1000 km pipeline connects them to the Atlantic Ocean at Kribi, on the Cameroonian coast, from where crude oil was shipped for export to refineries. Most of the pipeline's route lies in Cameroon. COTCO managed the operation and maintenance of this pipeline on Cameroonian territory.

We were also building offices in N'Djamena, the capital of Chad, this time for the headquarters of the production company EEPCI – Esso Exploration Production Company – a Chadian subsidiary of ExxonMobil, responsible for the exploration and management of the oil fields. This project was more advanced and the construction site was in its final phase. Once more I was responsible for the budget and making sure the project ran smoothly, something which had been particularly stressful.

To the question "why have offices in both N'Djamena and Douala since it's actually the same project?" the answer was simply: "Chad is not Cameroon". The Cameroonian government received dividends on the operation of the pipeline according to the flow and would have never agreed to administrative management being located in Chad.

Over the last two years I had commuted a lot between N'Djamena and Douala, using a plane – a Dash – chartered by our company, which made the connection twice a week; the two cities are 1000 km apart.

MOUNT CAMEROON
It was early November 2006 and I was in Douala, Cameroon. My wife Wanda was joining me there a week later with Edyta and Dominika, two Polish friends, for a short holiday. During the weekend of 11–12 November, we were going to attempt the ascent of Mount Cameroon (4040 m). We had been planning this mini expedition for some time.

Mount Cameroon, the highest peak in West Africa, the tenth largest summit of

Africa (the largest being Mount Kilimanjaro, 5895 m), was still an active volcano. It was actually the most active volcano in West Africa with nine eruptions during the twentieth century, the last one occurring in 2000. Thanks to preventative evacuations, those eruptions had never claimed any victims. The ascent did not present any major difficulties as it followed a hiking trail. It was the hot and humid climate that made things difficult. Rainfall on the slopes of Mount Cameroon was among the highest in Africa, with a record 14,655 millimetres in 1919. Because of the humidity we could hardly ever see this mountain from the city of Douala, located just 60 kilometres away. The sky was almost always hazy.

We departed from the city of Buea, located 870 metres above sea level on the east side of Mount Cameroon.

There were ten of us in the expedition. Besides Wanda and her two friends, there were my colleague Jean-Michel Tolen, his wife Désirée and Danièle Diwouta, an architect, with three of her friends, all Cameroonians. Jean-Michel had organized a guide and two assistants to carry the food. The guide was called Adolf: Cameroon was a German colony until the First World War and one of its colonial legacies was Cameroonians with German names.

The climb was more painful than expected. Although there were no really difficult passages, the slope was rough and the constant hostility of the volcanic terrain, consisting of hardened lava, gravel and holes, made the ascent very difficult. After 2000 metres, at the end of the rainforest, the trail climbed vertically, without zigzags – the "Wall" – in a savannah environment, to the second refuge located at 2800 metres.

It was a gruelling and poorly planned ascent. We should have taken three days but the professional constraints of some of the team members left us only two days to try to accomplish the impossible. When the rain started our hopes were dashed. We gave up at 2800 metres and spent the night in the second refuge, a stone cabin, tired and shivering with cold. That night part of the team tried to reach the third refuge, at 3700 metres, but most gave up after twenty minutes because of the lashing rain and came to find us at around midnight. Only Dominika, one of Wanda's Polish friends, continued with the guide Adolf who was probably less than enchanted by her persistence. They reached the third refuge and gave up, defeated by the wind and the icy rain.

The guides had prepared a picnic lunch with chicken sandwiches. The chicken

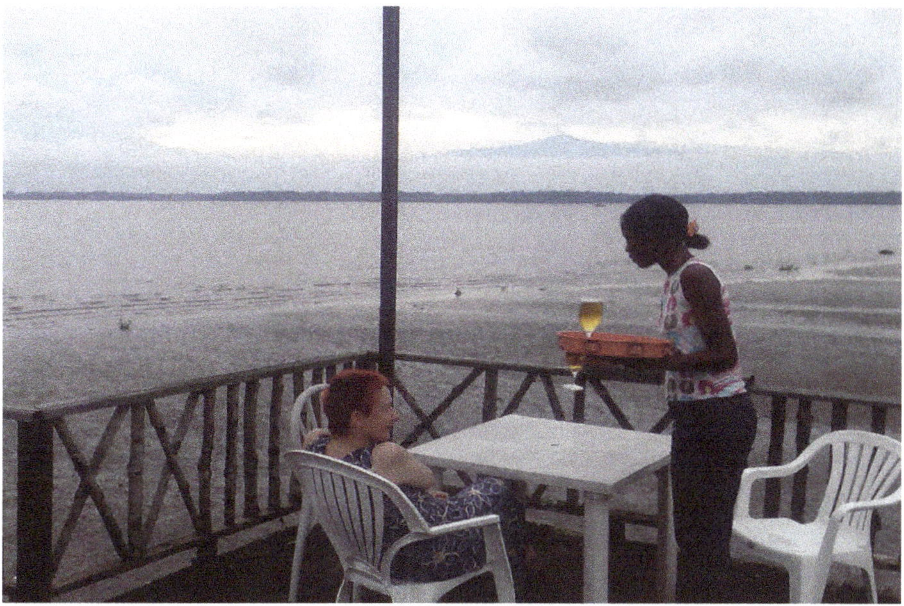

Mount Cameroon in the background, in the clouds, seen from Douala. A beer for our friend Dominika who just arrived from Poland.

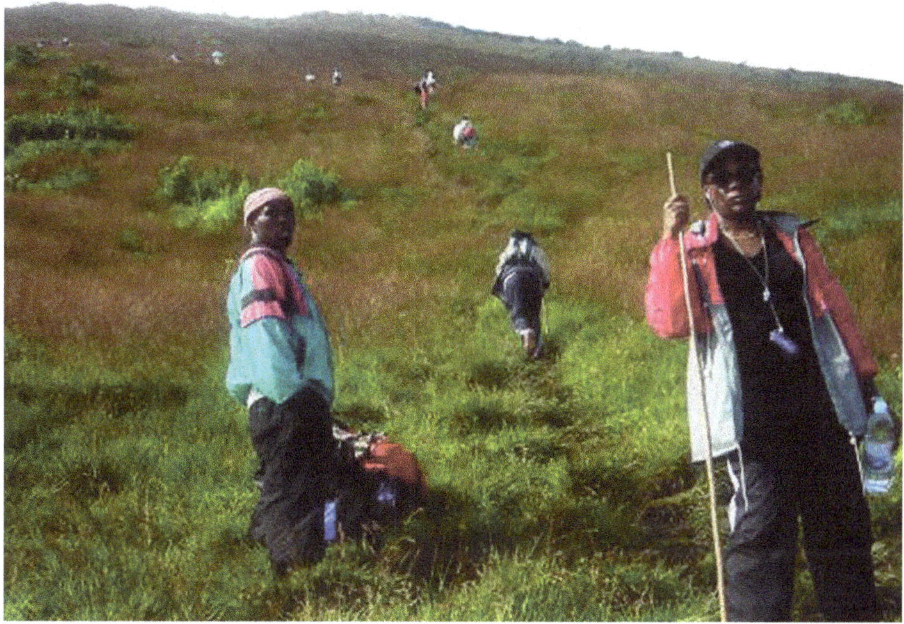

Ascending Mount Cameroon

© Désirée Tolen

was so badly cooked, with blood on the bone, that Wanda and some of the others refused to eat their share. I was so hungry that I did not mind and guzzled greedily. The night was bitterly cold, I could hardly sleep.

The descent the next day was also difficult. As we say in Switzerland "oh, oh! My knees". In the middle of the descent, we met a Cameroonian athlete who was training for the race up Mount Cameroon which takes place every year in March. Clad in shorts, he was climbing fast: impressive stuff. My legs were hurting and I didn't step back to let him pass until the last moment. He still had enough energy to bawl me out because I was in his way. I gave him a mouthful in return. Later, I felt bad, my tiredness had made me talk nonsense.

Our arrival in Buea on Sunday afternoon was a great relief. The last kilometre of the descent was particularly painful, I could no longer feel my legs, my knees hurt, my feet were blistered, I was covered in sweat and unable to talk anymore. The rest of the team didn't look too bad and nobody noticed the state I was in. Fortunately, the vehicles to bring us back to Douala were waiting for us.

The runner arrived shortly afterwards, fresh as a daisy. I had wondered whether he went to the top or stopped at one of the shelters. Apparently the best runners reached the summit in four hours. I didn't dare ask him in case he recognized me and got angry again. Actually, it was stupid of me to think that, the guy was very calm, happy to have done his run and just a little tired. A true professional.

The next two days, at work, my legs throbbed, my muscles ached. It was obviously the lack of training that had handicapped me, but I thought that maybe my age, 57 years old at the time, didn't help either. My colleague Jean-Michel, 20 years younger, who did not train and is quite stout, was also suffering but not as much as me. He hardly even had muscle ache. Wanda, who has had more training than me thanks to all her hikes in the Alps, was less afflicted. After the climb, she spent two days resting at the beach in Kribi with Edyta and Dominika. While I had to work...

AMSTERDAM
Thursday November 16, I flew back from Douala to the Netherlands for a week's
holiday before traveling to Nigeria for my new mission. Wanda had left the day
before. During my stay, I suffered from a slight "tourista" which started in the
plane to Amsterdam. I blamed Swiss, the airline, which must have fed me badly.
This was not my first gastroenteritis, it happened quite often and I did not pay too
much attention to it. Usually, I stopped drinking coffee, ate rice and it went away
after 2 or 3 days. But this time it lasted longer. This diarrhoea was also different
from the others I've had: darker, with a stronger smell (sorry for the details).
I thought it was weird but did not really worry about it. I didn't have stomach ache
or feel uncomfortable. I thought that I would have got rid of it by the time I left for
Lagos the following week but it was still lingering.

LAGOS, SUNDAY AFTERNOON NOVEMBER 26, 2006
In my hotel room, I relaxed with a DVD that I bought the day before in a small
market: the Lekki Market, or "Jakende" for the locals.

I knew this market and had visited it before. It was located on the outskirts of
the city, not too far from the hotel, about 20 minutes by car. I got driven there in a
company car.

The company did not allow expatriates to drive themselves: too many risks.
Instead, there was a pool of chauffeur-driven vehicles (Toyota Prado 4x4). We
just needed to call the central, identifying ourselves, tell them where we wanted
to go and they picked us up. But sometimes you had to be very patient as they
could take more than an hour to arrive, either because of the frequent traffic jams
or availability problems. I remember when, during a previous visit, I had wanted
to eat at a restaurant: after waiting in vain for an hour and a half, I resigned myself
to eating at the hotel. The car was stuck in traffic. But there was no more than 400
metres between the fleet and my hotel!

Nigel, my South African colleague, introduced me to this small market that
had a little bit of everything. As there were no tourists in Lagos, it was mainly
frequented by locals, apart from the occasional expat, like me. There was no
harassment. You could walk quietly in the narrow alleys, which were lined with
rudimentary stalls with corrugated iron roofs. That day, I was the only white
person there, but that did not bother me. Nobody payed any attention to me,

at least not obviously. It was very different from some North African markets where you cannot have a second of peace. Nigel had shown me a small shop that sold cheap DVDs, illegal copies of films from America and Asia for 1 dollar each. Nigel regularly came here to buy some and he brought them back to South Africa for his family. The first time I went there, a month before, I bought a number of damaged DVDs. It was now my second visit. The seller recognized me and when I considered a particular film he told me: "Don't take this one, it is not good", not to inform me that the film was third-rate but rather that it was a bad copy.

I watched the movie Stoned (2005), a comedy drama chronicling the last months in the life of Brian Jones from the Rolling Stones, which asked whether his death in 1969 was murder or suicide, without really answering the question. By the way, it was not a bad film. The image blocked five minutes before the end but I miraculously managed to restart it after a while by pressing "reset", "restart" and see the end. Phew.

But when I wanted to get up afterwards, I noticed that it was difficult, my legs felt weak. "I am very tired, I need to rest," I said to myself and went to the hotel restaurant for dinner. I would have liked to have eaten somewhere else but the thought of having to call a car and wait with no idea when it would show up put me off the idea.

Before going to bed, I tried to do some push-ups. I knelt on the floor. To my surprise, when I leant on my outstretched arms they collapsed under me. I crashed to the floor, almost breaking my nose. There was no strength in my arms. "I'm really very tired" I said to myself. But I felt no pain and decided to go to bed.

Alone in bed unable to sleep, I gave in to onanism, as many do without always admitting it. Nothing special except that I saw this time that the enjoyment was not accompanied by ejaculation. Dry pleasure? A bit surprising, but I thought no more about it and fell asleep, satisfied nevertheless.

MONDAY MORNING NOVEMBER 27, 2006
The hubbub of the nascent traffic on Lekki Expressway and the accompanying sound of horns penetrated the double glazing, pulling me out of my sleep at around 6 am. In any case, it was almost time to get up. I got out of bed, went to the bathroom and sat on the throne to relieve myself. I noted with dismay

that I could not get up again as I had no strength in my legs. It was really weird, especially as I was not in any pain. I felt stunned and unsure of what to do. I redoubled my efforts to get up but it was impossible. I managed to get on all fours and dragged myself to the bedroom. I put my elbows on the bed and managed to push myself up. Somehow, I got dressed. By this time I could walk again easily, so I went to the restaurant for breakfast and sat down at the table near the entrance. But when I tried to get up again after breakfast, I found that I couldn't, even when I leant my arms on the table. I resolved to ask the waiter to give me a hand to help me up. He complied and smiled, probably thinking what a feeble old man I was.

"THIS IS WHAT I THINK"

At the office, I immediately went to the company clinic located in the basement. After a short wait, Dr. Dominic Ukpong, the company's doctor, received me in his office. When I explained what had happened, he made me go to the auscultation room and sit on a high bed, where he checked my blood pressure and reflexes. He did not seem to find anything abnormal. We went back to his office and I sat in an armchair while he finished his auscultation report. When he asked me to get up, I couldn't. He got annoyed, thinking that I was playing the fool. I assured him that I really could not get up. Irritated, he called a nurse and asked her to bring a wheelchair.

They kept me at the clinic all morning, lying in bed, accompanied by the nurse. At some point, I wanted to go to the bathroom. It was a high bed and I managed to stand up. I took a few steps when suddenly my legs collapsed under me and I crashed to the floor. The nurse panicked for a moment, totally taken by surprise before rushing to help me up. She assisted me to the bathroom before escorting me back to bed. Fortunately, I was not hurt by the fall.

My colleague Samuel came to inquire about my condition. We were supposed to meet one of the construction company candidates for the renovation works, but I asked Samuel to postpone the meeting as I would be unable to attend. I explained that I did not know what was wrong with me and that I was awaiting the rest of the consultation.

Later that morning, Dr. Ukpong reappeared with a colleague doctor whom he had asked for a second opinion. They auscultated me, asking me to lift my arms and legs and testing my reflexes. They then spoke together in a low voice, without saying anything to me. The doctor nodded and said: "This is what I think". Then they left.

I laid on my bed, abandoned to my fate, with no information and no idea what was happening to me. But I did not feel any panic. I had no pain at all and kept telling myself that it was only a brief glitch and everything would get better soon. I was filled with an optimistic fatalism. The nurse was so kind and sympathetic to me. She got emotional, exclaiming: "This is not fair". I felt that she wanted to do something to help but was powerless, on the verge of tears. I ended up comforting her, reassuring her that everything would be fine. She then picked up a syringe and tried to take a blood test. All she managed to do was to butcher my arm, probably by lack of experience. It was a totally irrational action, as if she was trying to exorcise a demon that had taken hold of me.

At the beginning of the afternoon, she came back to inform me that I was being transferred to a clinic.

REDDINGTON HOSPITAL, VICTORIA ISLAND
Upon arrival at the clinic, I was given a lung X-ray as part of the admission examination before being moved to a private room. I could no longer stand and the nurse had to help me get through the examination.

A little later, I received a visit from a neurologist, a young, extremely beautiful Nigerian woman in her thirties. One of the ways she tested my reflexes was by stroking a feather along the soles of my feet.

She then said to me in a friendly but very assured voice: "We know what you have. Do not worry, you'll get better."

That simple sentence filled me with optimism. She had just told me that I would heal. It was fantastic news.

I did not know how long it would take, she did not say, but I told myself that it could hardly be a matter of weeks or months before I got better. She continued: "We could treat you here. But the treatment requires plasma that we do not have here. It must be brought from Europe. So it's better for you to go there."

Then I received a phone call from João Alves, my London-based boss who had been informed of my situation:

"Paul, you have to get out of there as soon as possible. You can't stay in this country with what you have."

I replied: "João, do not worry. They know what I have and have said that I'm going to get better, it's not so urgent."

He stated: "No, no, you must leave as soon as possible. I will talk to Dr. Ukpong".

I agreed.

Shortly thereafter, my colleague Adekunle Ali (Kunle) from the maintenance department came to see me. He told me that he knew the neurologist who had examined me and assured me that she was very competent. She worked in another hospital and had been brought here especially to examine me.

"Do not worry, you will get better": the neurologist's words resounded in my head. They were to give me courage throughout the ordeal that lay ahead.

Dr. Ukpong came to see me that evening at around 7 pm. He sat on a chair next to my bed, stared into my eyes with a serious expression and said: "We have organized your repatriation. You will be evacuated to Geneva tomorrow morning on a special plane. It was too late to do it today". This confirmed what the people in the hospital had already told me off the record. Repatriation is organized by SOS International, the insurance company contracted by my company. I heard later that they could choose between Johannesburg, London or Geneva. They opted for Geneva, saying: "He is Swiss, he must go to Geneva".

The night dragged on interminably. The night staff were chatting noisily in the next room and I could not get comfortable. To my shame, I needed help to go to the bathroom. Sleep eluded me.

TUESDAY MORNING NOVEMBER 28, 2006
My colleague Andy arrived early in the morning. He had collected all my personal belongings in the hotel room and packed them in my little suitcase. He arrived with a big smile on his face, saying: "This is Nurse Andy". I had always liked Andy and his resolutely optimistic character.

I had also received a phone call from the company nurse who inquired about my condition. I told her that I was OK and about to be evacuated. It was comforting to be surrounded by so many caring people.

I was told that I would be taken to the airport in a municipal ambulance instead of a private one as only municipal ambulances have direct access to the tarmac. I didn't quite understand the nuance or why they must explain this to me. For me an ambulance is an ambulance. Looking back, I think they just wanted to tell me that the clinic's services would stop as soon as I left the premises.

Before I left, the clinic staff joined me in my room. All five of them stood around my bed and wished me well. Nigerians could be so sweet.

My colleague Kunle came to see me again just before I got into the ambulance. I told him about the visit from the clinic's staff and asked him if I should have given them a tip, as I was so touched by their kindness: after all, tips are common in many African countries. He said: *"Of course not, they are just doing their job"*.

I still was not in any pain. The words of the neurologist the day before gave me courage. I knew that I would soon be better and able to walk again: I just didn't know how long it would take. The entire situation felt surreal. Other people seemed to see my situation differently and were obviously worried about my condition: after all, you didn't organize an evacuation for nothing.

I was accompanied in the ambulance by a young Nigerian doctor in a white coat. While the vehicle made its way through the traffic, revolving light on and siren at the ready, the doctor struck up a conversation with me. He scarcely inquired about my condition, but was more interested in working conditions in Europe, what he would need to do to get there and if I could help him. Lying on a bed–stretcher, almost unable to move, I just told him it was complicated.

LAGOS AIRPORT
The plane finally arrived and the ambulance set off towards it. I was taken out of the ambulance and put down on the bare ground, lying on my stretcher bed, at the foot of the plane: a Cessna chartered by SOS International arriving from Gabon. Later I was told that the aircraft was the property of Mr Bongo, President of Gabon. This was not really surprising since Mr Bongo apparently owned half the country. I am not sure whether this story was true, but most things have a sliver of truth somewhere. On board there was a doctor and a nurse, both Gabonese.

The pilot and the co-pilot were French.

It was time for the Nigerian doctor to hand over the papers documenting my case to the Gabonese doctor. As one spoke only English and the other only French, I had to translate the papers myself, lying on my stretcher on the tarmac. It was not too complicated as I knew what was wrong with me. I was paralysed, but I didn't know the name of the disease that the doctors thought was affecting me.

A Nigerian employee got angry: "Why don't they speak English?" The doctor calmed him down, telling him that they came from another country and therefore spoke another language.

It was time to get on the plane. No easy task when you can't walk. They put me on an inflatable bed, a kind of air mattress with high edges, which got stuck in the door. They had to fold it in half lengthwise, sandwiching me like a hot dog. It took four people to do this and hoist me up the stairs, through the narrow door and into the small plane. They put me on the floor, which had appropriate medical equipment. I would remain lying on this mattress for the entire flight.

My passport had meanwhile been returned, duly stamped. I was pretty relieved, as it had been gone for a long time. Then it was the pilot's turn to get upset, as he was still waiting for the flight authorization to turn up: "I gave them a bag full of money and still they do not return with the papers". He was worried that we would arrive too late in Geneva airport, which used to close at 10 pm. The plane had to go on to Paris afterwards.

After what seemed like an eternity, the documents finally arrived and we were able to leave. We took off just after 2 pm. As the flight lasted seven and a half hours, we were set to reach Geneva just before 10 pm.

The flight passed without incident. I was pretty well settled, lying on my back, but I couldn't turn on my side. At least I could stretch my legs when necessary. The doctor took my blood pressure every half hour throughout the flight. I was terribly hungry but did not get anything to eat. Maybe I needed to fast for auscultation on arrival. It became painful, especially when the crew and my companions started to eat. But at least I had an appetite, which had to be a good sign. The flight seemed to last forever and I couldn't sleep.

GENEVA

It was dark when we landed in Geneva shortly after 9 pm. From there, everything went very quickly. I was whisked away in an ambulance which left immediately without waiting for the customs formalities to be carried out. I barely had time to say goodbye to my companions. Hardly ten minutes later I was in a hospital. Less than one minute after that I was in the emergency department, in a room that resembled an operating room, lying on my back on what had to be a bed, with four masked faces bent over me. "Sorry for the masks, but you come from Africa, so as a precaution we must protect ourselves from possible infections" said a male voice with a Genevan accent. "I am hungry, can I eat something?" "Yes, but not right now, we must first do a lumbar puncture". I did not know what this was, so I was not too worried. I just felt as if I was in a bad dream in some endless corridor. Tired and starving. They turned me on to my side and I felt a needle penetrate my back ...

The pain turned out to be quite bearable, probably due to the local anaesthesia. I submitted without resistance, praying for it to be over soon. It actually went pretty quickly and it was a big relief when it was over. I was left lying on the bed, hoping I could soon have something to eat.

After 10-15 minutes they came back and said *"sorry, it did not work, we will have to do another puncture..."* What was this? A bad joke? But as I had no choice, what could I do except accept the situation and submit? I was just too tired to react and said nothing.

The second attempt was successful and afterwards, it was finally time to eat.

CHAPTER TWO

LA TOUR

"You have a Guienbaré". "A what?" "Guienbaré is a disease of the peripheral nervous system. We will treat you with plasma, it will slow down the disease and stop its development". That I understood, it is what I heard in Lagos.

One of the nurses in charge of intensive care explained things to me the day after my admission to La Tour Hospital in Meyrin, near Geneva. The test results were back and he wrote down the name of the disease for me: "Guillain-Barré".

He added: "Do not look for information on the Internet, as it's not verified and sometimes incorrect".

Lying in my bed I could hardly lift my arms or my head, but I still had the use of my hands. Cushions were placed behind my back to help me sit up a little. After a few days, I was able to sit on a chair with a tray, so that I could eat and read a little during the day. But I got tired very quickly.

GUILLAIN-BARRÉ SYNDROME
Guillain-Barré syndrome: disease of the peripheral nervous system (the nerves), following a deficiency of the immune system, symptomized by flaccid paralysis (flaccidity).

Guillain and Barré are the names of the two French doctors who identified this syndrome at the beginning of the 20th century.

They explained that after an initial phase of aggravation, the condition stabilizes, followed by a slow phase of improvement. The worsening phase is critical because it could affect the respiratory system, with fatal consequences:

later I would find out that 15% of cases are lethal. Plasma treatment with intravenous drip helps to check and stop the aggravation. After that there is no prescribed medication, the only treatment is physiotherapy.

This information was very encouraging. I was convinced that I would be totally cured within a few months.

My tests had revealed a bacterium: "Campylobacter Jejuni". This bacterium could be the cause of my disability. Although there is no scientifically proven correlation, apparently this bacterium is found in 30% of Guillain Barré cases. More importantly, it is found mainly in raw milk, cat excrement and undercooked chicken.

Badly cooked chicken... Dammit! But that's it of course, the undercooked chicken on Mount Cameroon, the second refuge, at 2,800 metres. The red chicken on the bone that others refused to touch and that I ate despite everything, tired, cold and starved. This was the cause. Bingo! For me this seemed obvious, beyond reasonable doubt. I caught this disease from that poultry! I swore that I would never eat chicken again. Never, ever again.

Dinner arrived and what do I see on my plate? That's right: a chicken leg. What would I do now? As I was ravenous, I resigned myself to eating it. I approached the chicken carefully, turning it in all directions, ensuring that it was well done and there was no red blood on the bone. Finally I swallowed it, slowly, in small pieces, leaving it to fate and praying with all my heart that nothing happened...

The head of the clinic, a Genevan in his forties with a very marked accent, (the same voice as the mask, when I arrived) introduced himself: "Do not worry, you will get away with it. I have a friend who had this a few years ago and now he is fully recovered. He loves the mountains and he is frolicking on the trails again like a kid, just like he used to." These words were very encouraging, they corroborated those of the Nigerian neurologist as well as the information provided by the nurse. My optimism rose even higher. Once again, I was convinced I would be restored to full health in just a few months.

An assistant also told me that the Lagos Hospital had produced an excellent report: "We should congratulate them".

Later, I was made to understand that there could be lasting consequences, that they could not promise me a 100% recovery. "In some cases, patients have to use a cane for the rest of their life" my brother told me during one of his visits, after making inquiries. But this kind of information did not affect me too badly, as I thought that it didn't apply to me.

INTENSIVE CARE

The two days of plasma treatment were difficult. The treatment itself wasn't painful, it was just an intravenous drip. A bag full of plasma hung from a vertical stem, a bracket, and a tube connected it to my left arm's vein. But meanwhile, the disease had progressed. Fortunately, I was not in any pain, but I was almost totally paralyzed, barely able to lift my head. I lay on my back and couldn't even turn on to my side. I could move my arms but couldn't reach the bell hanging thirty centimetres above me. At my request, one of the nurses brought an extension cord and put the bell next to my pillow, within reach. This bell was important, it allowed me to call for help when necessary.

And it was then that the ordeal begun. I could not sleep. I was uncomfortable. I wanted to change position constantly but couldn't. I rang the bell to call the nurse on duty to ask her to help me turn to one side and then the other. This went on all night. I think I had to call them at least fifteen times. Sleep was impossible. I needed a sedative, a sleeping pill, but couldn't have medication when I was on the intravenous drip. In tears, I asked them to sit me at a table and put a pillow on it so I could lean over it with my arms around it. And that's how I finally found a little rest, sometime around 5 am. What kind of demon has taken hold of me?

After two days, once the treatment was over, I was given morphine, which helped me to sleep a little better the following nights. "Minimum dose" assured the nurse in answer to my question, "not enough to become addicted, do not worry".

Apart from the inconvenience of not being able to move, I do not remember having suffered during this period. My wife Wanda reminds me, however, that I complained about pain. Maybe muscle pain? Maybe that's why I could have morphine? It's still a total blank.

FIRST VISIT

It was during this initial intensive care period that Wanda and her son Sebastian flew from Amsterdam to see me. Although I was happy to have them near me, I was exhausted and asked them to leave me alone after about half an hour as I had no more energy to talk to them. This seemed to surprise them. They spent one night in Geneva and returned to Amsterdam the next day, as scheduled.

Sebastian told me much later that he had been shocked by how ill I looked. My throat was very swollen, as if my muscles were no longer holding it up. I could not move. Cushions supported my back and head, lifting me into a half-sitting position. Wires and pipes connected my body to various control screens and devices. I must have looked dreadful. I did my best to tell them that this was only temporary and I would soon be better. I have no idea if they were convinced.

EMILIO

It was not long before my father Emilio came to see me all by himself, even though he was almost 99 years old at the time. He arrived in a taxi from La Tour-de-Peilz, 80 kilometres away. It must have cost him a fortune. I did my best to welcome him, smile and express my optimism. I think that this first visit was a relief for him, that I looked better than he had imagined. He couldn't see very well and I think he didn't quite realize the state I was in. Neither did I for that matter.

My brother Raymond and my sister-in-law Marie-France who lived near Lausanne, drove up to see me once a week, stopping in La Tour-de-Peilz each time to pick up my father. It's a long journey.

INTENSIVE CARE STAFF

I have unbounded admiration for the nurses and assistants who cared for me during that intensive care period. What infinite patience, care and devotion. Never a derogatory remark, not even after the fifteenth call that night. Always smiling. These people were heroes.

One nurse used to come and massage my back. She did it very gently and lovingly. It wasn't just a quick rub: the massage seemed to go on for hours but was probably ten or fifteen minutes. That woman was an angel.

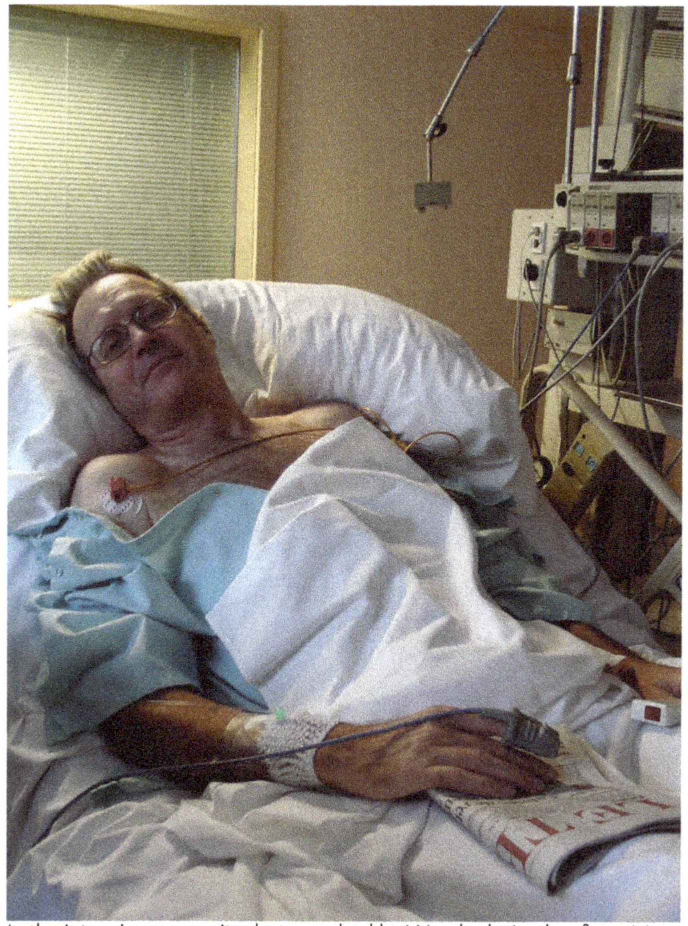

In the intensive care unit, photographed by Wanda during her first visit

© Wanda Michalak

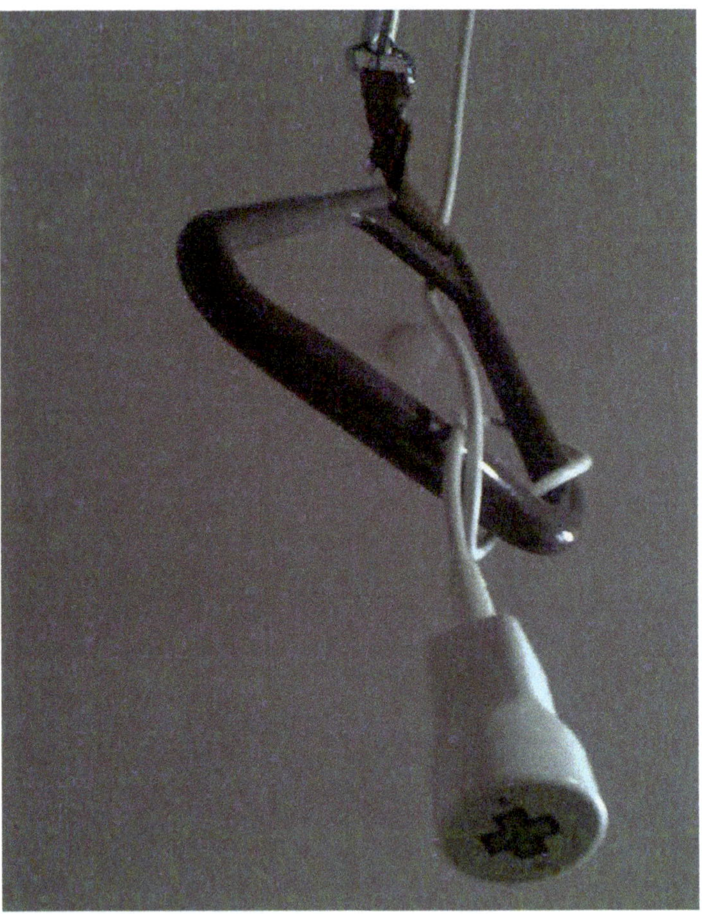

The unreachable bell, hanging 30cm above my head

CONTINUING CARE

After two weeks, my case was no longer considered critical and I was transferred to follow-up care. I was entitled to a private room and could start physiotherapy. By this time, my condition had slightly improved and I could manage, albeit with great difficulty, to turn myself around in bed, which allowed me to sleep better without having to call for help all the time.

The intensive care nurse who had told me about Guillain Barré came to see me. He sat down beside me and told me about a motorcycle accident he had been in a while ago, his injured arm and the time it had taken him to recover. His nerves had also been affected. He explained that my damaged nerves were recovering very, very slowly and that it would take many months or even longer for them to heal. All this was to let me know that I would need to be patient as I would not heal overnight.

Through the window, I could catch a glimpse of the Jura mountains. The sky was grey and overcast. This gloomy weather, typical for the month of December in this part of the world, would persist throughout my stay in this hospital. As I never saw the sun, I had to look for it in my heart and tried my best to do so.

NEW ALERT

Two days after my transfer to follow-up care, I noticed a tightness in the left half of my face, which I reported to two medical assistants during their morning visit. They looked alarmed and left hurriedly without saying anything. They thought it looked like the beginning of facial paralysis. They were right. I was having a relapse. I immediately underwent a new plasma treatment. My face continued to deteriorate rapidly to the point where I could hardly speak.

I had a moment of intense panic. Not because of my situation as I remained resolutely optimistic about my prospects. I was worried about my father: if I could no longer speak it would be impossible to reassure him about my condition and he would be sure to panic. His next visit was scheduled a week later, together with my brother and sister-in-law. I called him on the phone while I was still able to talk to tell him that everything was fine and I was looking forward to seeing him again next week. My voice was still audible. I felt that my condition was getting worse and I prayed that it would improve before next week.

For two or three days my condition continued to deteriorate. My mouth was all twisted, half paralyzed. A speech therapist, specializing in communication disorders, made me do speech exercises "a" "e" "i" "o" "u" "ou" "en" "on", etc. To be repeated several times, very loudly. She gave me several sessions and speech exercises to perform on my own.

She was a funny lady, in her fifties, with dark, medium-long, curly hair. She had a sad, unenthusiastic face with drawn features, as if she was always tired and weary. She was neither motivated nor motivating. "Menopausal effect?" asked my wicked subconscious. Well, maybe having a job where you have to constantly ask patients to say "a" "e" "i" "o" "u" was not very exciting.

Fortunately, the new plasma treatment had the desired effect. After three days my condition had improved noticeably, as if by magic. The facial paralysis had virtually disappeared by the time my father came to visit.

ELECTROMYOGRAPHY

I also had to undergo electroneuromyography (ENMG). A specialist was called in to measure the conductivity of the nerves in my legs, to try and assess the damage and confirm the cause. The exercise involves measuring motor nerve conduction velocity (MNVC). He chose my left thigh for the examination. He stimulated the peroneal nerve above the knee with a brief electric shock and measured the response of a distal muscle that was part of the motor territory of the stimulated nerve in the upper thigh. The shock was extremely brief and I did not feel any pain, not even a tingling.

This guy was also a strange character. He was a skinny, bearded, forty-something with dark greasy hair in a side parting and a funny, high-pitched voice. He reminded me a little of Kees van Kooten, a Dutch comic, in the role of the "vieze man" (old pervert). He talked to me while doing the tests, complaining that he was not allowed to work as he would like, that he would have liked to have conducted further tests. I don't remember exactly what his problem was, but my lasting impression was of a terribly frustrated man. By that time, I was wondering what the point of these tests were. He told me that everything seemed OK, that the nerve was there. But I never heard anything about the results.

I now understand that this examination made it possible, among other things, to distinguish a peripheral neuron lesion from a primitively myogenic lesion (attack of muscle fibres). In my case, it was done to confirm that what I had was a neuron peripheral injury and that we were dealing with Guillain Barré syndrome.

This examination can also have a prognostic effect if it is repeated several times to follow the evolution of the syndrome. But this was not done for me. Maybe that is what the specialist was complaining about.

I observed that, between the electromyographist and the speech therapist, I was surrounded by people who were not very motivated. Instead they seemed depressed and exhausted. Fortunately their intervention in my case was only very sporadic.

That was in such a stark contrast to the young intensive care team, who impressed me with their enthusiasm and motivation. Perhaps their activities are less routine and require more initiative.

PHYSIOTHERAPY

There was no medication for Guillain Barré syndrome. The only treatment in the "recovery" phase was physiotherapy, to recover use of the affected muscles as far as possible.

The physiotherapist in charge was Sandrine, a Genevan in her thirties. She was very dedicated and extremely enthusiastic. She made me perform daily exercises, which were limited due to my severely diminished functionality. Every day I had to breathe into a device to measure lung capacity. This was a routine test to check whether my respiratory system was functioning properly. The physio sessions began for real by moving from the bed to a wheelchair. This required the assistance of a nurse as I was practically a dead weight, unable to lift myself. The exercises consisted of trying to lift my legs, weight training with dumbbells, (I could barely lift 500 grams) throwing balls, leaning forward and trying to get up, etc.

After a few days, Sandrine brought me to the indoor pool. She lowered me into the water on a platform suspended from a winch. Once in the water I noted with astonishment that I could move my legs and practically walk in the water. "You see?" she said, "your limbs are working, you can walk, everything will come back little by little." I was speechless. What an amazing moment to see and feel

my legs working. It was incredibly encouraging. A sublime moment. I did not want
to stop. I could walk in the water! I wanted to exclaim, "Long live Archimedes"
although that did not really make sense. I had discovered hydrotherapy. Sandrine
was also extremely enthusiastic.

THE STEEP SLOPE

I was at the top of a mountain looking down. The slope was steep, covered with
tall grass that bends under its own weight as it undulates in a light breeze. It's
weird grass, very thick and soft, a greyish-white colour with brown spots here
and there. In fact it was not grass and there was no wind. Looking closer, I realized
I was looking at chickens. Hundreds, thousands of chickens, alive, packed tight
against each other, busy pecking. They formed an imposing febrile mass that lined
the steep slope as far as the eye could see, like a very thick carpet. I rushed down
this slope effortlessly and in slow motion, striding, bouncing cheerfully every
five to six metres, barely touching the thick, feathery carpet. It's as if I was gliding
through the air, weightless. Lower down, there was forest and flat open country.
I saw myself slowly disappearing in the depths below, leaping gently without a
hitch, until I was only a tiny point on the horizon evaporating in the mist. It was
such a sublime feeling of tumbling down a slope, easily and smoothly.

I woke up in my bed, delighted to have had such a pleasant dream, while
disappointed to be once more in my difficult present, lying almost paralyzed
in bed. But that dream was encouraging, loaded with optimism, it gave me a
good feeling. It was to stay with me. The experience of the pool, having seen my
legs move, undoubtedly counted for something. And this mountain was Mount
Cameroon. And the chickens ... Yes, I will walk again! I want to! I can!

THE CHAD POWER GENERATORS

During one of his visits, my brother Raymond told me about his discussion with a
doctor friend who suggested that what had happened to me could also be linked
to stress. This is an interesting comment as I had been very stressed for an entire
year before my accident.

A memory of a particularly hellish night in N'Djamena, Chad, a year ago, came
to mind. A problem with the generators had been keeping me awake at night.

We were in the midst of renovating and expanding the offices. Due to budget constraints, we decided not to replace the two old generators which had just about enough capacity to meet demand. Even worse, we could not afford to add a reserve (the N+1 as we say in technical jargon).

The frequency and especially the length of power cuts of the city's only power plant had been underestimated. A second power station was scheduled but construction was far from complete. It would therefore be necessary to resort often – much more often than anticipated – to generators to operate the building. On one visit, a power cut lasted more than 48 hours. I watched anxiously as the two coupled generators blew and vibrated, ready to give up the ghost at any moment. And the building was not yet being used to maximum capacity as extension works were still in progress.

There was a real risk of an inexorable generator failure, which would have resulted not only in impossible working conditions – it's impossible to work without air conditioning when the average outdoor temperature is 38 degrees Celsius – but also in the loss of computer data as the backup batteries only lasted 120 minutes.

To top it all off, the client was threatening not to accept the project until the problem had been solved. He told me at a meeting that he preferred to stay in temporary rented premises, with all the ensuing financial consequences. I felt terribly responsible.

I remember the sleepless night that followed that meeting. The problems swam round and round in my head and reached a paroxysm. There was no one to talk to and I felt like banging my head against the walls. I was alone in a miserable room in Tréguer, the guest house. It was impossible to adjust the fan coil (it was either "off" or "on" and the "off" was not an option) so it blasted out cold air above my bed, causing an unbearable draught that forced me to wrap myself up in the blankets. There was a TV but the programmes were useless and I could not concentrate anyway. Even Sudoku – a sort of crosswords with numbers instead of letters – which normally forced me to concentrate and allowed me to escape my thoughts did not help. I almost shouted in despair, I could not see any way out, I was in an endless tunnel. Alone in the middle of the night I had no one to talk to or confide in. I ended up having a very loud cry and screamed at the top of my lungs. This calmed me a little.

The next day, at the office the problems had been put into perspective. After all, they were only technical hitches which were solved a few weeks later when a request for additional budget was granted, making it possible to acquire the missing generator. The customer agreed to occupy the new premises in the meantime, the allotted delivery and installation time of the additional generator being six months. But meanwhile, I had been scarred and subjected to terrible stress.

I probably still was: having to manage three projects in three different countries simultaneously was extremely stressful. I did not blame anyone, however, as it was my choice.

This explanation made a lot of sense to me. It was possible that this stressful situation affected my nervous system and contributed to my immune system dysfunction. Surprisingly, no one else had mentioned this factor. Neither in Nigeria, nor at La Tour Hospital, nor at the rehabilitation centre that I went to later.

THE VISITS

I received several visits during the five weeks I stayed at La Tour Hospital. In addition to the aforementioned family members, there was my boss João Alves, who came especially from London to see me: a one-day flying visit that honoured me. He too was shocked by the sight of me. Later on, he was to tell me that he thought I would never be able to go back to work. He stayed two hours with me. I could see his thoughts ticking over: he had to find a replacement for the three projects I was responsible for. But this visit had made it clear to him that he could not count on my return in the short term, or maybe not even in the long run. I was unable to talk to him about it, the very thought of it stressed me out. And anyway, what could I say? I think he intuited this and did not press me on the matter. I got on well with João, I appreciated the trust he put in me. His mentality (he is Portuguese) and opinions were close to mine. We spoke French together. João was very familiar with Africa, having spent several years there. He had worked in Congo-Kinshasa as the company's national director, so he understood the specific problems we were constantly facing: slow implementation, imports and customs problems, associated logistical problems, etc. He often said, "Our management in Houston, they understand nothing about Africa, we cannot explain it to them". He was also a very kind person. He told me once how, in Congo, he used to buy monkeys sold on the street (monkey meat is a delicacy there) and released them back into the wild.

I later found out that three different colleagues were going to take over the projects I had been forced to abandon: Paul Begnaud in Lagos, Jan Kerremans in Douala and Nora Belobrk in N'Djamena.

My old university friend and partner-in-crime, Nabil, also visited me. I really appreciated his visit, knowing how much he hated hospitals. We were soon to meet again in a totally unexpected situation.

My friends Jean-François, Yves and his wife Anne-Lise came to see me from Vevey. Yves was particularly shocked when he put a bottle of wine in my hand and my arm sagged under the weight. He caught it just in time before it crashed to the floor, exclaiming "oh well, okay". It would have been a shame, as it was a nice Vaudois vintage Corseaux, if I remember rightly, that I appreciated to the full a few weeks later.

All these visitors must have been horrified by my appearance, but no one ever let me know.

I received phone calls from many friends in Holland, where I lived. Gerrit: my soul mate; my old friends Mees and Marianne; Christie; Hannie and Wouter from Toulon. I remembered the command from Wouter, Hannie's new companion "Paul, promise me never, never, never to return to Africa".

Everyone thought I caught this disease in Africa. This was not true: this disease hardly exists in Africa, it occurs mainly in the so-called developed countries. My illness manifested itself in Africa, but this was pure coincidence. I could have been anywhere.

DIGNITY
The entire hospital staff was kind and friendly towards me. Most of the people I came into contact with, had lived in France and crossed the border every day. The only Swiss people taking care of me were the head doctor, my physiotherapist and the peculiar electromyographist and speech therapist. More than 50% of the hospital's employees must have been foreigners. How on earth would it have operated without them?

One of the things that stuck out in my mind was trying to retain some dignity even though I had to rely on my caregivers for everything. I could not wash myself, and every time I needed to go to the toilet, I had to ask for help. It took two nurses to lift me out of bed and put me on the loo. If you could not wash yourself, you had to get used to being naked in front of other people and letting them wash your private parts. I didn't mind so much with the female nurses, but I felt rather awkward with the men. But I had to accept the fact that I was dependent on these people. What choice did I have? Actually, it was funny how quickly you get used to things and stop worrying about them.

For the first five days of my stay in hospital, I was unable to pass a motion. This worried me terribly as I thought that the weakness of my intestinal muscles was disrupting the peristalsis of the digestive tract (progression of the alimentary bolus from the pharynx to the rectum). I was scared that this situation would never right itself. Imagine the relief when I finally managed to produce a tiny poo. I had been so embarrassed by all the times I had mobilized an armada of assistants to carry me to the loo, only to be unable to produce anything. Thankfully, this situation was temporary and my fears were unfounded.

There was a somewhat peculiar nursing assistant, a little man in his forties with a Near Eastern or Eastern accent (I have forgotten his nationality), who once commented on the size of my mini droppings when he emptied the pot. One day he was taking me to the toilet, supporting me by the buttocks, when he "accidentally" slipped a finger into my anus when lifting me. I was so surprised that I did not say anything. I will never know if he had done it on purpose or if it was an accident. I strongly suspected the first option, but what could I have done? Accused him? Called the head nurse and told him that the guy "fingered my ass"? After that, I was on my guard whenever he came near me, but there were no more incidents of this kind. This episode serves to illustrate the state of total dependence and vulnerability inherent to my situation.

CONFIDANT
Over the weeks, I became Sandrine's (the physiotherapist) "confidant". She was on the point of splitting up with her husband and would tell me about her marital problems during our daily sessions. She used to pick me up in my room, transfer me to my wheelchair, guide me through the corridor and take me through my

simple and often repetitive exercises, all the while updating me on the latest developments in the crisis. Sandrine needed to pour out her heart to someone and I was a good audience, listening and nodding from time to time. Maybe I was the ideal audience: unable to escape and compelled to listen. I didn't mind my new role at all, on the contrary. I couldn't give her any advice as I didn't know her husband and was clearly unable to judge the situation. Anyway, I don't think that that's what she was after. She just needed to unload her grief, as is so often the case in this type of situation. I felt kind of proud of being chosen to act as her confidant. It made me feel normal again, to be more than just a useless patient: in a way it gave me back some dignity.

Sandrine's relationship was a real saga. Sometimes the situation improved and she and her husband would go for a meal together and talk. During these periods, Sandrine was full of renewed hope. These truces never lasted long and sooner or later the fighting would resume. One day, towards the end of my stay, Sandrine informed me that they had decided to separate. She did not look sad: on the contrary, the decision seemed to come as a relief to her. It was just before Christmas, and she was about to go on leave. That was the last time I saw Sandrine, as I was being transferred to a rehabilitation centre. I will never know how things turned out for her, whether they broke up for good or embarked on a new round of reconciliation efforts.

During one of our last sessions, Sandrine arrived in tears. She had just heard that a patient whom she had become very fond of had died. She was devastated. The relationship between patient and physiotherapist can be very intense. Sandrine and I spent thirty minutes to one hour together every day. Over time, we became close, you could even have called it a kind of intimacy. We got to know each other as we talked and exchanged ideas. I experienced that feeling not only with Sandrine but also with other therapists during my recovery process.

THE TUNA

One day I was having lunch in the hospital restaurant with my father, brother and sister-in-law. I was seated next to my father, in my wheelchair. Raymond and Marie-France had gone to the self-service buffet when my meal arrived: a plate of tuna. My father was in the middle of a story, so I took a bite of fish. I probably bit off more than I could chew as it got stuck in my throat. I started coughing.

Blissfully unaware, my father carried on with his story. I panicked, unable to breathe. Choking, and unable to make a sound, I tried to get my father's attention by gesticulating wildly. My father remained oblivious to my plight as I gasped for air, flailing my arms around. Suddenly, the head doctor rushed out of nowhere and slapped me hard on the chest and back, eventually managing to dislodge the tuna. He intervened just as I thought that I was about to suffocate. The doctor left as abruptly as he had arrived, without saying a word. Meanwhile my father had finally noticed that something was not quite right, so I told him what had happened. When Raymond and Marie-France returned carrying their full trays, they were amazed to hear that such a dramatic event had occurred during their absence. The entire incident had lasted less than two minutes.

It turned out that I had been inadvertently served a fat-free meal intended for a heart patient. I now understood why the tuna was so dry and difficult to swallow. This goes to show that accidents can happen in no time flat. I was incredibly lucky that the doctor saw what was happening and knew exactly what to do.

SOS INTERNATIONAL
Christmas was coming, and I had been in hospital for four weeks. The head doctor arrived and announced: "We can't keep you here any longer. You are no longer in a critical condition, the worst is over. It's time for you to go to a rehabilitation centre". I said I wanted to rehabilitate in Switzerland, somewhere close to my father if possible.

However, my insurer wanted to repatriate me to the Netherlands, where I lived, as health care and treatment is much more expensive in Switzerland.

I was not very pleased by this prospect. I wanted to stay in Switzerland, my home country, close to my elderly father, in a familiar environment. Wanda agreed with me, saying: "You will be treated better here than in Holland". I told João, my manager, who conveyed the message to our management in Houston. Nick Greco, manager of the ExxonMobil Global Real Estate Group to which I belonged, contacted SOS International's director whom he knew personally. It was finally decided that SOS International, our company's insurer, would remain responsible for my case until further notice so that I could continue treatment in Switzerland.

Sandrine recommended the Valmont centre in Glion-sur-Montreux, eight kilometres from La Tour-de-Peilz, city of my childhood where my father was still living. I jumped at the idea, as going back to my roots felt like the right thing to do under those circumstances. Valmont confirmed that a place was available and I could go there just after New Year.

THE HOLIDAY SEASON
As the holidays approached, the head of the clinic informed me that they had decided to provide a Christmas meal for my entire family at the hospital and asked how many of us would be attending. This unexpected gesture touched me deeply.

There were thirteen of us at the table. Besides Emilio, Wanda, Raymond and Marie-France, there was also my niece Sabine and her boyfriend Afrim, my nephew Eric, my other nephew Robin with his wife Mary and their daughter Cléo, and Concessa Denervaud, a friend of the family, with her sister. An almost biblical assembly.

The three-course meal was absolutely delicious and we could drink as much wine as we wanted. They really treated us well. A secluded place had been organized in a corner of the restaurant and we had the space to ourselves. My nephew Robin even congratulated me for choosing such an original venue.

I was so happy to have my family and friends around me. I almost felt normal again, until Wanda asked me to open the small bottle of eau de toilette she had given me, but my hands weren't strong enough to open it. This brought me down to earth with a bump.

I was extremely grateful to the hospital for allowing this meeting and organizing it so well.

Wanda stayed in Switzerland and came to see me on December 31, along with our friend Gaby and a bottle of champagne. They left around 6 pm, leaving the rest of the bottle with me. By 9 pm I was nicely tipsy. The duty nurses noticed but turned a blind eye. I fell asleep well before the twelve strokes of midnight. A surreal end to the year.

CHAPTER THREE

VALMONT

*The walker up the Montreux Hill inevitably stops in front of Clinique
Valmont, three quarters of the way up the slope, seized by the
beauty of the building and the mystery that emanates from its
elegant and silent mass in the trees. It is a fin de siècle building,
in the style of the composite palaces that made the bay famous.
A long, three-storey, flat-roofed building, at the centre of which
stands a kind of kiosk, or extravagant cottage. The whole rests
on a glazed ground floor, finished by a column rotunda lined with
Virginia creeper and lily.*
 - Jacques Chessex - extract of his novel La Trinité.

"Your condition is serious. You will have to consider moving to somewhere with fewer stairs". The head doctor was speaking to me. His tone was quiet, monotonous and severe. He was in his fifties, quite tall and thin, with slightly greying black hair in a side parting. He was sporting a little moustache, glasses and his medical white coat was unbuttoned. Either he had not introduced himself when he entered my room, or I had not been paying attention. He was accompanied by a silent assistant whom I had seen two days earlier when I had been admitted. I came to understand that was to be the first of the head doctor's routine bi-weekly visits (the "medical parade" was the name given to it by a Dutch "comrade in misfortune" whom I later found on the Internet).

"Who was this bird of ill omen," I asked myself. "And how did he know that my house has stairs?" But he was right. Our small, narrow house in the centre of Amsterdam had three floors and no lift. I did not answer him and he did not stay long: there was not much to auscultate, my case was clear and he had read my records.

I wasn't bothered by his pessimistic comments as I was still buoyed up by the encouragement I had received in Geneva and Lagos. I was convinced that I would recover quickly and soon be as good as new.

THE CLINIC

My arrival in Valmont two days earlier on Tuesday, January 2, 2007, had not been very cheerful. January 2 was a depressing day anyway, when everyone had to go back to work after the holidays. The weather was grey and cold. I was taken into the building via the service entrance at the rear, through the gangway between the imposing building and the steep slope of the mountain that leads directly to the second floor. "You are late", I was told. "It is after 11 am and new admissions are always before 10 am at the latest." The small, edgy man in a white coat talking to me was the doctor in charge of admissions. With his square head and wide mouth, he looked a little like Tim Robins, but the comparison stops there. He had a stern look about him and if he had a sense of humour, it was very well hidden. His tone was unpleasant, even unfriendly. His rapid speech and "lack" of an accent betrayed his French origins. "One of those little, nervous, frustrated ones," I said to myself. He accompanied the head doctor on the medical parade. I listened to him, wondering how on earth he could blame me for being late. It would have made more sense to complain to the friendly paramedics who had driven me from Geneva but they had already left. Eventually I was admitted: after all, they could hardly leave me sitting in the corridor in my wheelchair! I did not know then that I would spend nearly 5 months in this establishment.

The Valmont Clinic was very different from the Geneva Hospital as it is a rehabilitation centre specializing in neurological and orthopaedic rehabilitation. Everything there was more humdrum and scheduled. Many of the patients were victims of cerebral strokes with neurological damage (partial paralysis, loss of speech…), "cardios" (cardiovascular accidents or heart attacks) or they had broken limbs in serious accidents. The average age of patients was quite high, especially in the neurology section where I was placed. At 57 I was among the youngest. I assumed I would be the only case of Guillain-Barré as it was such a rare disease, but I soon learned that there was another case in the clinic, a lady, whom I was to meet a few weeks later.

A ROOM WITH A VIEW

My room was located on the second floor. Once more, I had a private room complete with a bathroom and a balcony, thanks to my employer's SOS International cover. "How nice! And what a wonderful view from the balcony. "You can see Lake Geneva and the surrounding mountains", exclaimed Wanda. "A room with a view". It sounded idyllic, almost like a scene from The Sound of Music. A dream place to recuperate. But as far as I was concerned, it was no use to me, confined to my bed. All I could see from there was the sky. I could not manoeuvre my wheelchair over the threshold to the balcony, and when the window was open I could hear a constant background noise that seemed to come from far away. It was the hubbub of the motorway traffic on the viaduct at Chillon some 150 metres below. It reminded me of a muted version of Piccadilly at rush hour. Noise pollution is not what I would call romantic. Fortunately, the windows were double glazed and since it was winter, they were closed most of the time.

Wanda travelled between Holland and Switzerland to visit me. She came once by plane and twice by car, accompanied by a friend (she did not want to drive the 1,000 km from Amsterdam on her own). She stayed in our small chalet at Le Trétien in the Valais Alps, 40 minutes away from Valmont. Wanda was apprehensive about driving in the mountain but the situation didn't leave her much choice. She actually got used to it quickly and this gave her more confidence behind the wheel. At least something good was coming out of this situation.

NEW ROUTINE

I soon settled into a routine, consisting of two or three daily sessions of physiotherapy and occupational therapy except at weekends. Each session usually lasted thirty minutes and was given in the basement. Later I would also have hydrotherapy in the indoor pool on the same floor, where there was a beautiful view of the garden from a large, south-facing window. Lunch and dinner were served in the large, stately dining room on the ground floor.

I was wheelchair-bound for exercise and meals. The first few days there was someone to push me but I soon managed to fend for myself as there was just enough strength in my arms to propel myself forward. At first I was very slow and nearly everyone overtook me. I began making it a point of honour to pass at least one of the stroke patients who were struggling to walk with a stick along the long, wide corridor leading to the dining room. But I was frustrated when orthopaedic patients with broken legs or feet sped past me in their wheelchairs. I tried to push harder but in vain. Too slow! There was a young mountain climber in his twenties who had broken both feet in a rock-climbing accident. He got up to speeds of at least thirty kilometres per hour in his wheelchair. He was like a Formula 1 driver. Maybe the effort helped him to unwind. Another patient, Fernand, in his forties, had broken both legs falling from a horse. Although he was not as fast as the mountaineer, he was not far behind. One of his legs jutted out in front of him horizontally, protruding from his wheelchair. I was constantly afraid that he would bang it into a wall, a door or a person and break it all over again. Luckily Fernand was very nifty and good at avoiding obstacles. We were soon to become friends.

At first I needed help to get into my wheelchair but after three or four weeks I managed this by sitting at the edge of the bed and slipping onto the wheelchair on a rigid plastic board that the physiotherapist had given me. It was a strenuous, time-consuming operation as I did not have enough strength in my arms to lift myself and was only able to slide centimetre by centimetre. The first few times, I managed to sit in the chair but the board remained stuck under my buttocks and I hardly had the strength to remove it. When I finally mastered the technique, my satisfaction was intense. Finally, I had regained a little bit of autonomy.

Breakfast was served in bed every morning at 7 am. Tea, toast, butter, jam and yogurt. Swiss breakfast is a good alarm clock. It was served very quickly and I didn't have time to say anything, especially as I was still half-asleep. During the first few weeks my hands were too weak to unscrew the lid of the jam jar so I had to ask the nursing auxiliary for help. Later I mastered this as well.

Between 8 and 9 am it was time to get washed. I was totally dependent on the auxiliary or nurse to take me to the bathroom and wash me, propped up in a chair. I had got used to this at the Geneva Hospital and no longer felt any shame at being so exposed and dependent. I was always treated with great respect and my dignity was preserved. These people were true professionals.

I was usually taken care of by Christophe, a young Frenchman who became my friend. One day he brought his PC so that I could upload hundreds of songs to my computer: the complete works of Barbara, Brassens, Brel, Renaud, Zebda, Noir Désir, Muse, and many others. Even today I have still not listened to all of it.

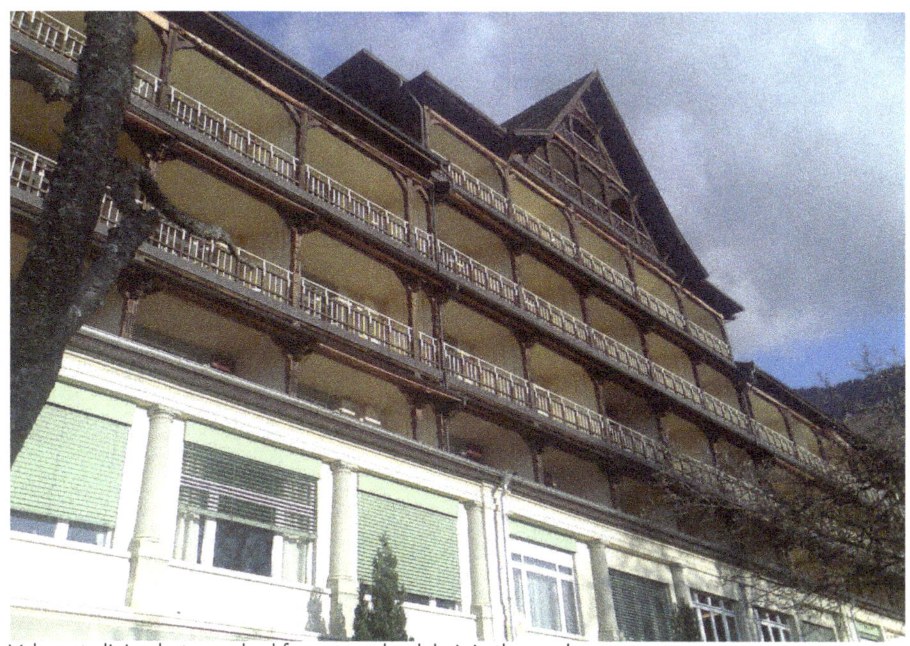

Valmont clinic photographed from my wheelchair in the garden

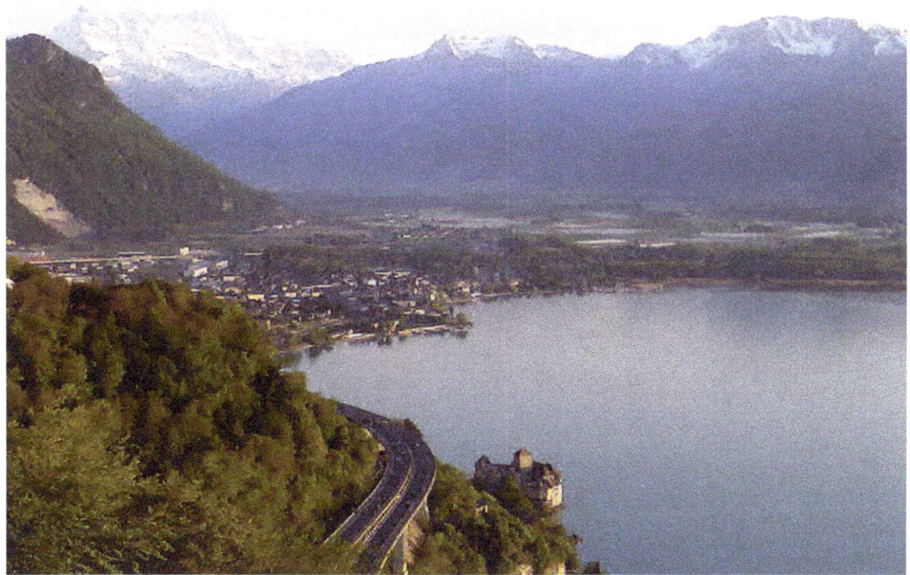

The view from my balcony, which I could only enjoy at the very end of my stay

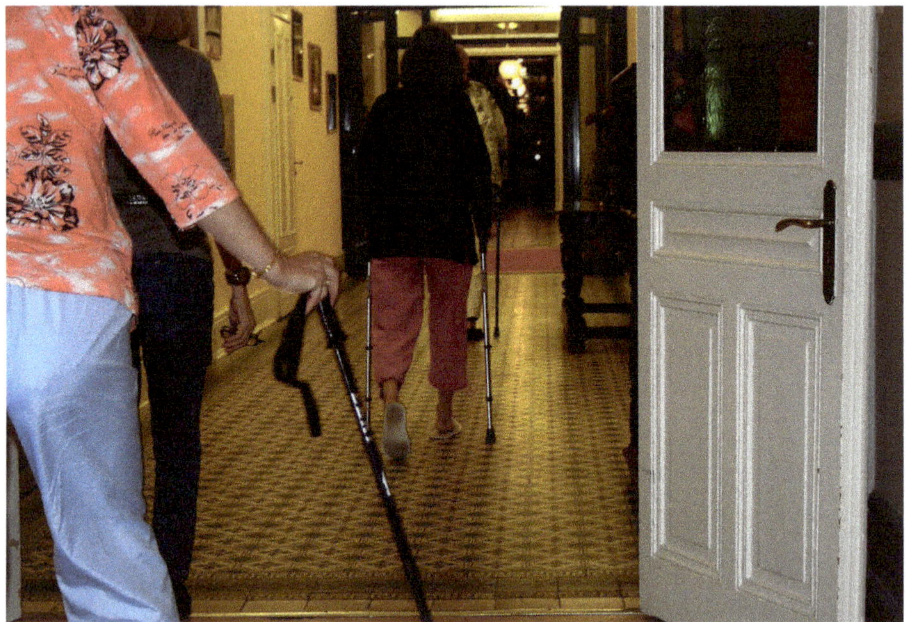

On the way to lunch © Fernand

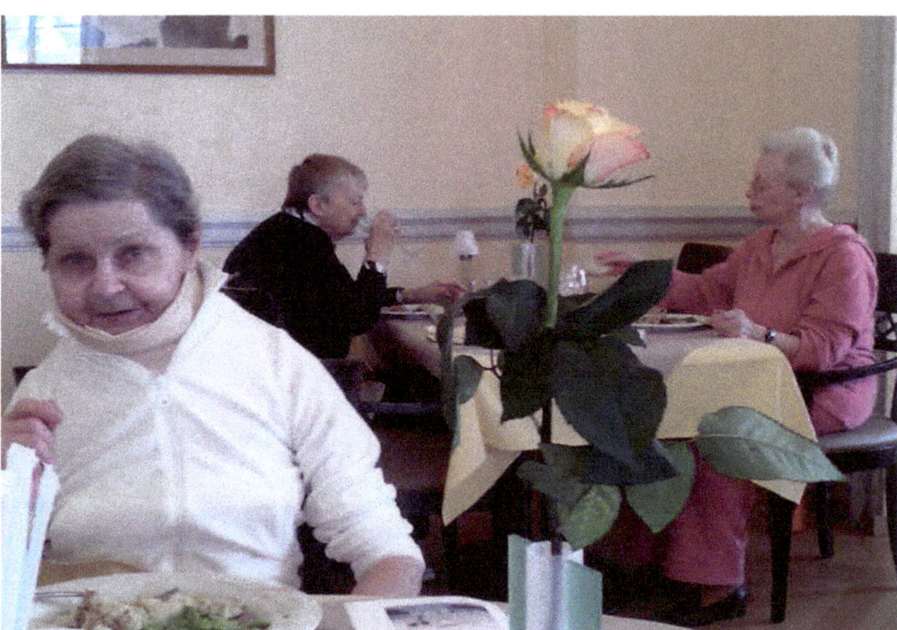

My table companion for a while

I had never heard of Muse or Noir Désir, and I'm still not convinced.

We both had to laugh one day when he lifted me off the bed to take me to the bathroom but had not brought the wheelchair close enough. Both unable to move, we clung to each other as if we were lovers. It had us in fits.

Sometimes I was washed by Amina [1] a young woman from the Maghreb. She was nice, kind, always smiling, with curly black hair and a beautiful round face. She used to give me a wonderful head massage when she washed my hair. Unfortunately she didn't take care of me often.

One fine morning Christophe and Amina both entered my room laughing, plonked themselves at the foot of my bed and asked me which of them I preferred to wash me. I was briefly taken aback, but I did not hesitate for long and stated my preference for Amina, "because she knows how to massage my head". Christophe looked piqued, did he really think I could have chosen him? How could he have thought that? The problem for him was that the alternative to me was a particularly difficult patient in the next room. He left without saying a word. This was when I realized that I was relatively popular with the employees.

At noon lunch was served in the large dining room on the ground floor. I had a place at a table by the window, lake side, overlooking the garden. It's a privileged place for private patients. The garden was lined with tall trees and bushes which obstructed the view of the lake and the surrounding mountains. I would have liked to have seen the Grammont, just across the lake, a mountain I had climbed twice in my youth. This mountain could predict the weather. If it seemed distant, it was a sign of good weather but if it looked close you would be sure that bad weather was on the way. I learned this when I was a scout. The meals were, moreover, excellent. They even served wine, usually from the region, reminding me that I was in wine country.

These were rather exceptional circumstances under which to return to my home country after an absence of more than thirty years (I moved to the Netherlands in 1975). Vevey, my place of birth, was about ten kilometres from Valmont. La Tour-de-Peilz, my father's hometown and where I spent a lot of my childhood, was even closer. I could never have imagined anything like this happening. Apart from my condition it was extraordinary to be so close again to my father, Emilio. In February we would celebrate his 99th birthday.

VISITS

My close family, my brother Raymond, my sister-in-law Marie-France and my nephew Eric regularly came from Lausanne to visit me on Sundays and picked up Emilio on the way. Many other friends also came to see me. My friends from my youth, Jean-François and Yves, who had already visited me in Geneva, Yaneth, the young Peruvian who took care of my father and lived in Montreux, Danièle and Pierre-André from Le Trétien in Valais, a visit I particularly appreciated.

Serge Wintsch, an old friend of my brother, also came. He was a jazz fanatic who organized the Jazz Onze Plus Festival in Lausanne, a small festival highly recommended by true jazz fans. [2] He brought me a stack of CDs including the complete Roland Kirk. I was amazed as he normally doesn't lend anyone his CDs.

My young niece Sabine came on Valentine's Day and I invited her to dinner. A special table was prepared for us in a corner of the large restaurant. I was as proud as a peacock to have her with me, especially on a day like that, and told everyone, "this is my niece".

To my surprise my old study mate Nabil came to see me with his wife Christina. This was his second visit after Geneva. I really appreciated it, knowing how much he hated such places. It was a cold but sunny Sunday in January. Nabil pushed me around the garden in my wheelchair, well wrapped up.

And then there was Nora who travelled all the way from Paris with the TGV for one day. She was our architect for the Chadian project and replaced me as project manager. Construction was now complete and she came to review the financial closure of the project with me. It was both a professional and a friendly visit. I observed her look of surprise when she noticed my hands trembling as I wrote. Although she said nothing I could imagine what she was thinking. For me it was a pleasure to see her again, as enthusiastic and optimistic as ever. She had not forgotten to bring the wooden school slate a Chadian artist had presented me with.

My condition was improving slowly but it must have been difficult for all these visitors to hide their concern about me. I tried to reassure them by adopting a positive attitude, which probably surprised them. Yet this optimism was sincere. I was convinced that I would recover in the long run so there was no need for people to pity me too much. I hated pity.

BOGOUSSLAVSKY

During her first visit my sister-in-law asked me if I had seen the famous neurologist, Dr. Julien Bogousslavsky. I had never heard of him. She explained that he had been head of the neurology department at the Lausanne University Hospital (CHUV) but had been forced to leave his post last year in the wake of a scandal. According to her he was now in Valmont.

I made a few inquiries and discovered that not only was this neurologist in Valmont but that he was in charge of me. He was the doctor who had stressed the seriousness of my condition and urged me to consider moving to a house with fewer stairs.

I was surprised to learn that he was an internationally renowned neurologist. Nothing about this shy, scowling man would have given you that impression. Even more improbable was the fact that he had masterminded a huge scam. When he was head of the neurology department at the CHUV hospital he had managed to embezzle more than 5 million Swiss francs. According to the press, it was a sophisticated scam that could only have been conceived by a brilliant mind. It was discovered purely by chance when an assistant stumbled across it.

Under arrest, Dr. Bogousslavsky confessed to his crime and apologized. He declared that he had embezzled the money to satisfy his all-consuming passion: collecting valuable art books. Fortunately he managed to auction off his collection for a good price and repay the misappropriated funds in full. After 8 weeks he was released on bail.

While awaiting trial in the summer of 2006 he was hired by the Valmont Clinic, just a few months before my admission. Prof. Bogousslavsky's professional reputation was invaluable to the clinic who wanted to use it to attract a wealthy private clientele including Russians. When questioned by the press, the clinic's manager asserted that the neurologist had not been assigned any administrative or accounting tasks.

I was intrigued by this man and fascinated by his criminal side. His outstanding intelligence; the subtle way in which he had managed to embezzle so much money; the fact that he had committed this crime for a "noble" cause, the love of art; that he had repaid everything: all this compelled a kind of respect, even admiration.

Moreover, being in the care of such an eminent neurologist comforted and in a way honoured me. From a medical point of view, I could not be better off.

His gloomy prognosis did not get me down: on the contrary, it encouraged me. I wanted to show him that he was wrong about me and that I would make a full recovery.

All these factors boosted my confidence and changed my attitude towards this serious, sullen man. He must have noticed it because eventually our relationship became more cordial. I even got the occasional smile out of him.

Dr. Julien Bogousslavsky's trial took place in 2010. He was finally sentenced to a two-year suspended sentence and a fine of 180,000 francs. Two years later he received an additional fine of 100,000 francs. The fact that he had repaid the money he had embezzled in full (5.3 million francs) and that he had no criminal record and a brilliant reputation kept him out of prison.

It turns out that Serge Bogousslavsky, Julien's father, was also an art buff with criminal inclinations. He had hit the headlines in Paris in 1939 for stealing l'Indifferent, a famous painting by Antoine Watteau from the Louvre in broad daylight. He returned it two months later explaining that he was in love with this work and that he wanted to remake the varnish and the framing, which he found appalling. Bogousslavsky senior was sentenced to 4 years in prison. Apparently, art-related crime is a family affair.[3]

OCCUPATIONAL THERAPY

The team of occupational therapists were great. It was composed of three women, two of whom, Catherine and Magalie, were French. Catherine was my regular occupational therapist. She was in her thirties, married and lived nearby. Magalie was from Thonon-les-Bains, near Evian and drove 60 kilometres to work, crossing the border at Saint-Gingolph, at the foot of Mount Grammont. She complained about the strength of the euro against the Swiss franc which at the time was around 1.5 francs for 1 euro. She must be happy now, since the euro lost in value.

Catherine made me practice dexterity tests for my hands and arms such as sorting scrap metal, pushing blocks on a board by stretching arms, stacking small cubes, raising my arms and passing objects from one hand to the other.

I progressed to standing exercises, held up by a strap in a sit-to-stand lift, a steel structure topped with a tablet to rest the arms. The device was kept in the corridor, so that you couldn't miss seeing it when entering or leaving. I compared myself to a pastor getting ready for the sermon. To spend time in this position I did puzzles. Though it didn't feel that way the occupational therapist programme was well thought-out. Each session featured a new challenge and all progress was meticulously recorded.

The occupational therapists formed a tight-knit team, sharing two adjoining rooms. Catherine and Magalie were very close, probably because of their nationality. They were always in a good mood, chatting and telling jokes. Sometimes they also told me about their lives. This created a pleasant and affectionately nonchalant atmosphere. This did not make them any less professional: they observed every movement, correcting me when necessary, giving encouragement and congratulations as appropriate. They always had the greatest respect for their patients' dignity. I appreciated this, as it would have been so easy to treat people in our position like children.

Sometimes, they were diabolically naughty and asked more intimate questions to test the patient's reaction. Once they asked an elderly stroke patient, paralysed and sitting in an electric wheelchair, if he had already cheated on his wife. He responded "Frankly, right now I do not have much libido, this question doesn't interest me." I felt exactly the same way.

I couldn't stop laughing when they treated themselves to a Chippendale evening in Montreux to celebrate a birthday.

Catherine was going on holiday to Amsterdam. I gave her my address and asked if she could maybe visit my home and evaluate it from an ergonomic point of view. Unfortunately, there was no one at home to let her in, but she could already see from the outside that the wheelchair would not be able to get through the front door. Also the height of the building meant a lot of stairs. She fell silent and that spoke volumes in itself. She seemed to agree with Bogousslavsky's opinion that I would need to move house. I felt spurred on by her response as this was one more reason to fight hard and make progress at any cost. I was determined to walk again.

PHYSIOTHERAPY

Physiotherapy was much more sober. Grégoire, my regular physiotherapist, was from the area. He was in his thirties, tall, skinny, with glasses and short, light chestnut coloured hair. He was always serious, devoted and concentrated. But we did not share any emotions or confidences. It was 100% physio. He started working with me in mid-January and we worked together for the rest of my stay in Valmont. At each session, he pushed me beyond my limits. He mostly worked on my legs, which were the worst affected by this blasted syndrome, by making me do pedalling, bending and weight-bearing exercises on fitness equipment. The main problem for him was getting me into position on the equipment. I was still so weak that he had to lift and carry me. He tried to make me walk on a treadmill, suspended in a harness. He often brought me to the pool for hydrotherapy. The process of transferring my virtually inert body weighing 70 kilo from the wheelchair to a winch-operated board was a strenuous task for him.

For the first two weeks, before Grégoire came, I had been taken care of by Solange [1], a French physiotherapist of West Indian origin. She contacted Sandrine, my previous physiotherapist in Geneva, to ask for more details about my condition. She tried to teach me how to get from bed to the wheelchair. She also made me do back-strengthening exercises in my room. One simple exercise was to lie on my back and try to lift my belly by making a bridge, leaning on my feet and shoulders. I had to repeat this exercise on my own. Although Solange was nice she did not seem particularly motivated. She talked a lot about herself and her forthcoming wedding. She told me about her passion for the animated films of Hayao Miyazaki and showed them to me. This was a whole new world for me and I watched "Princess Mononoke" (1997), which I managed to download by following instructions emailed to me by her fiancée. Technically, it was a beautiful film but it didn't really interest me. Maybe because my concentration was still under par. Although I didn't bother watching it to the end I was touched by the fact that someone who didn't even know me had bothered to send me an email telling me how to download it. I am not sure that I would have gone to so much trouble for a total stranger. Solange left two weeks later, she had handed in her notice. Maybe that's why she seemed somewhat unmotivated to me: she had made her decision and was probably counting the days until she left.

WORK

One fine day, I received a phone call from Jan Kerremans, a work colleague from Brussels. He was taking over the supervision of the Douala project in Cameroon and needed me to brief him on the project by phone. I asked him to contact me early in the morning, between 7:30 and 8:00 am, as this was when I could think most clearly, uninterrupted by my daily activities. Over the next two or three weeks, we had a series of early-morning conversations, sometimes followed up by emails. Having to talk about work made me nervous. It was not only for practical reasons that I preferred having these conversations early in the morning: I also wanted to be free for the rest of the day. The mere thought of having to work in the afternoon or even worse in the early evening or having to wait for a professional phone call was simply unbearable. This bothered me and weighed on my mind. In other words: it stressed me. The tsunami of questions, responsibilities and problems resurfaced, making me nervous. I wanted to forget everything, convinced that my illness was somehow connected to the demon of stress.

FIRST OUTINGS

Grégoire, the physiotherapist, had got the measure of me and I soon observed progress, especially in my arms. I could propel myself faster in my wheelchair.

On February 8, I made my first family outing to celebrate my father's 99th birthday. Catherine, the occupational therapist, made me practice getting from the wheelchair into a car. The trick was to stand with your back to the vehicle, sit on the side seat, legs outside the vehicle, then slowly rotate ninety degrees while tucking your legs in to get into the right position. Unable to stand on my own, I needed help to do this exercise.

My brother Raymond took care of the transport. We went to the Palais Oriental, a Lebanese restaurant in Montreux overlooking the lake. Raymond had inspected the premises to make sure they were wheelchair-friendly. There were eleven of us. In addition to the family (Emilio, Raymond, Marie-France, Eric, Sabine, Afrim, Wanda and myself), there was Yanneth, my father's companion and her husband Fred, as well as Iwonka, a friend from Amsterdam who came with Wanda. My first car outing was a success and there were more to follow in the weekends ahead.

On March 10 we celebrated my sister-in-law Marie-France's birthday in Pully, near Lausanne. My brother suggested that I spend the night at their home, as this would be more fun and also easier from a logistical point of view. It was a weekend and the Valmont team approved. My first night out of the clinic was an exhilarating step towards my liberation. My niece Sabine and her boyfriend at the time, Afrim, picked me up. Afrim, a sturdy Kosovar, carried me up the stairs to my brother's first-floor apartment. At least I only weighed 70 kilos. Even so, Afrim was exhausted when he dropped me on the sofa. I slipped from his arms and almost fell on the floor.

On Catherine's (the occupational therapist) advice, my brother had scrutinized his apartment, especially the door entrances and access to the bathroom to make sure that I could access everywhere in my wheelchair. He drew up a highly detailed plan as befits an architect.

It was a very pleasant evening. Marie-France had prepared traditional couscous, one of her specialties. The whole family was there, including my father and my nephew Eric. My second nephew Robin, his wife Mary and their daughter Cléo, then 5 years old had come from Zürich. Little Cléo was very impressed to see me in a wheelchair. She watched me, her eyes round, hovering between fear and curiosity, too shy to speak to me. Wanda was not there as she had to attend a preview in her gallery in Amsterdam.

I went to bed happy, but in the middle of the night I woke up, needing to urinate. I sat at the edge of the bed and reached for the vase meant for this purpose, which was on a small table nearby. Instead, I slipped off the bed and fell to the floor. I managed to satisfy my need, but could not get back into bed as my arms and legs were too weak. It was 5 am and I did not want to wake everyone. So I waited. I managed to pull the duvet over me, but I was uncomfortable and unable to get back to sleep. Around 7 am I took my mobile which was on the bedside table and called my sister-in-law who was sleeping in the next room. She and my brother quickly arrived and got me back into bed asking, "Why did you not call earlier?" "I did not want to disturb you in the middle of the night". Actually it was quite comical: phoning someone who was in the next room because I had fallen out of bed! I could see the funny side but it was probably very worrying for my family. I was still convinced that I would soon be back to normal and these inconveniences were only temporary. My daily progress reinforced this belief.

I went on several other outings in the following weeks. One Saturday my friend Jean-François took me to our chalet at Le Trétien. It was weird to be there in a wheelchair and I noticed the living room floor was not even as the chair started rolling by itself from the window towards the kitchen.

Some neighbours came to see me, but I felt embarrassed and no one knew what to say. I did my best to act "normally", to explain that I was making good progress and that I would soon recover.

Another time, Jean-François brought me to Vevey to dine with friends at La Valsainte, a restaurant near the school where we spent four years of our youth. I appreciated their consideration and the lengths they went to, to make sure I could get to the table in my wheelchair, with people getting up and moving chairs to let me pass. But what I appreciated even more was the fact that they disregarded my disability once I was seated. Being treated as an equal allowed me to forget about my situation and to feel normal.

On April 14, Sabine and Afrim got married in Lausanne. The entire Kosovar community was there, the women sitting together on one side and the men on the other. The highlight of the feast was a sheep's head. It was a festive and colourful evening that made us feel as if we were in the Balkans rather than in Switzerland. By that time I was able to walk tentatively, clinging on to the furniture. I even managed to sit on a bar chair. Little Cleo was there and stared at me, amazed to see me out of my wheelchair.

From then on, I spent almost every weekend at my father's apartment in La Tour-de-Peilz, where he lived alone. I was brought there either by a nurse who lived in Vevey, or by an acquaintance of my father. This was a win–win situation for both my father and I: he had company and I got to spend time in a normal situation. My father often said, "You are going up, I am going down". But he was incredible: even at the age of 99 he still had all his mental faculties.

CHRISTIANE WILKE

Towards the end of January, I met Christiane Wilke, a fellow patient who also had Guillain-Barré. She was 8 years older than me and came from Leysin, in the Vaudois Pre-Alps. She had been diagnosed with the disease about a month before me, in October 2006. It took a day or two for the staff at Monthey hospital to diagnose her with Guillain Barré Syndrome. Her symptoms were different from mine, mostly affecting her hands and feet. The paralysis in her hands must have been very trying. At first she was unable to hold a pen or even a knife and fork. For three months she could not feed herself unassisted.

We made friends and shared our experiences. There was a sort of friendly competition between us to see who could recover faster, which was encouraged by the occupational therapists. We started walking almost at the same time. As her feet were very weak, she had to use crutches.

I realized that the Nigerians had done a great job by diagnosing my condition straight away and making all the right decisions for my evacuation, especially as Guillain-Barré is not a common disease in Africa.

Christiane relates the onset of the disease as follows: *I woke up October 2nd, 2006 without being able to lift my knees. I called my doctor who recommended I go to the hospital. He arrived there at 4pm and immediately ordered my hospitalization. A neurologist was to examine me and since there was none at the Monthey hospital, the one from Martigny arrived at 7:30pm and diagnosed the illness. Then I had to undergo a lumber puncture. Two people failed doing it. The following morning a third nurse came to demonstrate how it is done. Well, she didn't succeed either. An anaesthesiologist finally managed after several tries and admitted it was not easy, my spine presenting a zigzag pattern! This resulted in a two-day delay to start the treatment which still had to be ordered.*

I noticed Christiane was very critical towards our chief neurologist. Among other things she blamed his lack of empathy. For example, at their first meeting after her admission for rehabilitation, he bluntly told her she would never recover the use of her hands. This was in the same trend as when he told me my case was severe and I should consider moving to a stair-free home. His policy obviously consisted of announcing the worst-case scenario and then hoping for the better. This might have been well-meant but in some cases such a brutal approach can deeply disturb a weakened person and one would have hoped for some more diplomacy.

Other incidents followed, like the sudden decision to end the use of morphine without warning from one day to the other. Probably a justified decision but brutal in its application, again affecting the sensibility of a patient who was unable to prepare herself psychologically for the change.

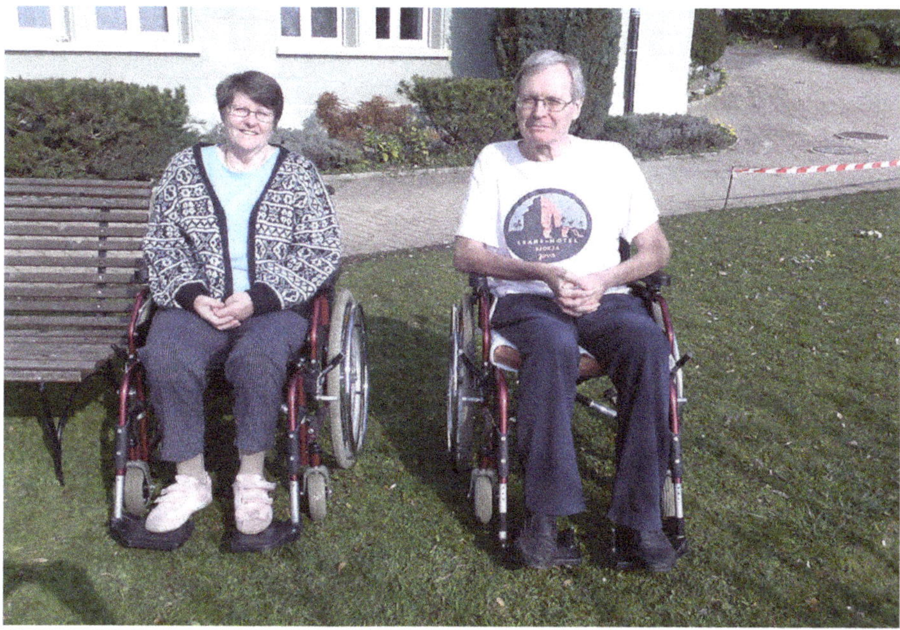

Christiane Wilke and myself in the garden   © Herbert Wilke

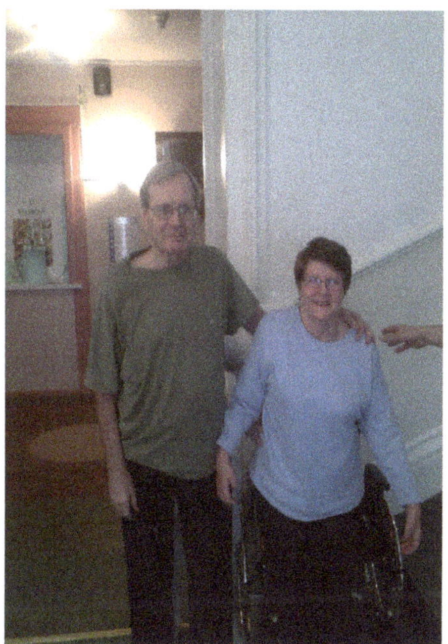

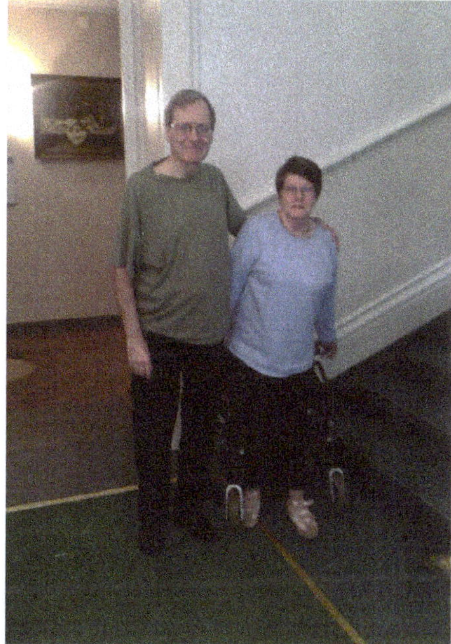

First photos with both of us standing, a big milestone

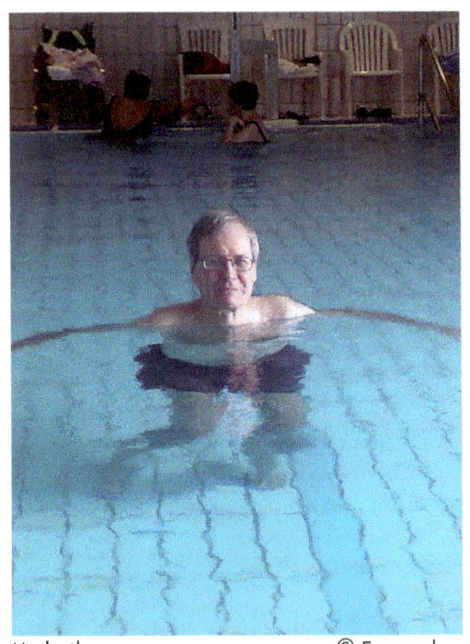

Hydrotherapy © Fernand

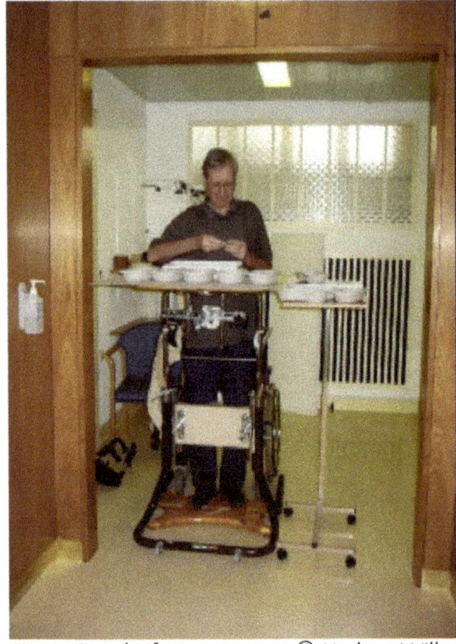

Sit-to-Stand Lift © Herbert Wilke

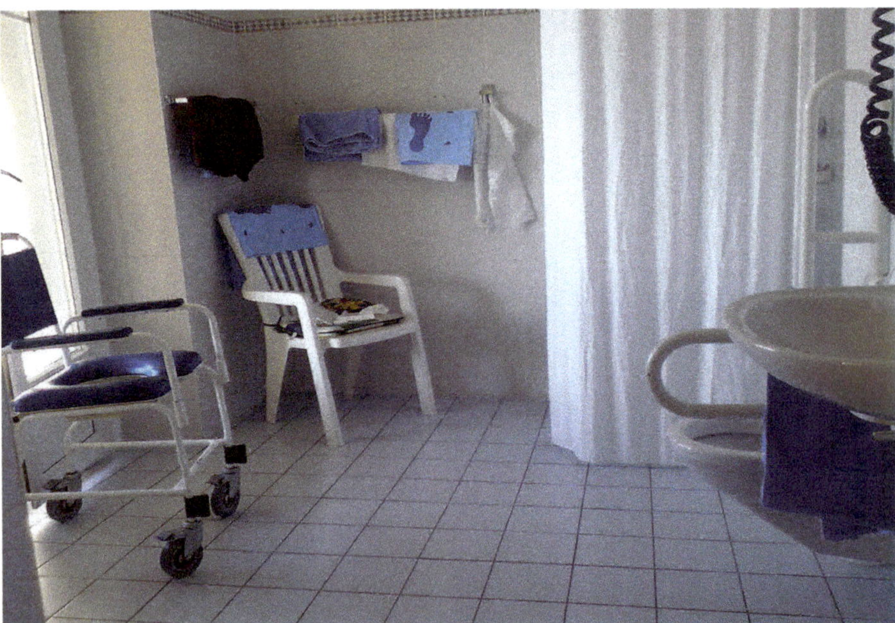

My bathroom, previously one of the rooms which hosted Rilke back in the 20's

When I met Christiane, four months after her hospitalization, she had partly recovered the use of her hands.

MICROCOSM

Around the same time I made friends with Fernand who had broken both legs after falling from a horse. In the dining room he invited me to join him at his table located in the back, away from the windows, which he shared with two other patients. "Come and eat with us, there is a free place and it's more fun than sitting all alone." It was only then that I realized that there was a hierarchy among patients according to their health insurance. The "private individuals", with extra cover were entitled to a place on their own, close to the south-facing bay window. The "common people", with only compulsory basic insurance, were seated in the back of the room and had to share their table. These seating arrangements also reflected whether someone had a private or shared room.

Fernand was a special case. He had been at Valmont for a good while. During this time he had become fond of some of the stroke patients and he encouraged them not to give up and to fight for their mobility. There were several very sad cases of people with cerebral strokes who were partially paralysed and sometimes even unable to speak. Fernand had a big heart and wanted to help. He took an interest in me when I explained what had happened "Wow, that's unreal," he said. I reassured him saying "Do not worry too much about me, I will recover. It is nothing compared to some stroke patients who have dim prospects. In a way you and I are both privileged". To kill time Fernand started to photograph everything happening in the clinic. He prowled the corridors, the kitchens, the physiotherapy room and the occupational therapy room in his wheelchair, his camera slung around his neck, one leg jutting out in front of him. He also photographed me doing my exercises at the pool.

There was a retired acoustic engineer, a heart patient, who told us that he was an authority in the field of acoustics in French-speaking Switzerland. He told me how he had been hired as a consultant by the Montreux Jazz Festival after the Stravinsky auditorium had been selected as the new concert hall (the old casino had gone up in flames in the 1970s). As the name suggests, this auditorium had originally been designed for classical music, not jazz. There was not much time for consultation, as the premises had to be ready in time for the next festival.

He described the terrible pressure exerted by Claude Nobs, the festival organizer, and his almost dictatorial attitude. He used to phone every day to monitor progress and stress the need to make the deadline. Obviously a lot of money was at stake.

The consultant confirmed that additional retaining columns were needed to properly contain the ground vibrations caused by the amplified bass sound. The balcony chairs also needed upholstering. The work was finally completed on schedule. They must have done a good job because the auditorium's acoustics are outstanding.

I asked the engineer what he would do to solve the problem of the noise pollution caused by the constant traffic on the Chillon viaduct. His answer was simple and radical: "Nothing". He continued: "We cannot do anything, the noise will only increase. The only solution is to insulate the windows". But the windows were already double glazed and the only way to soundproof the balconies would be to enclose them in glass; an expensive, unsightly and impractical solution. We would just have to put up with the noise.

There was also a lady in her forties from Romont, in canton of Fribourg, who managed a gas station. She had broken her leg and hip in a serious traffic accident. She was extremely popular and had lots of smiling and friendly visitors. I bet her station did very well. One day she introduced me to a representative from Esso who had come to visit her as we were working for the same company. The following year she sent me a nice note after my father died. She had read the notice in the local newspaper and remembered my name. This little note touched me. What a kind person.

Another patient was a nice woodcutter from the Jura who had half his foot amputated because of gangrene. I did not know that there were still such extreme cases of gangrene in Switzerland.

I also shared a table with a Serbian patient who had taken Swiss nationality. He was in his fifties and recovering from a heart attack. He liked to talk about how he was hoping to maintain sickness benefit until he reached retirement age. I do not remember exactly what his job was, but apparently it was not very interesting.

One day, a septuagenarian heart patient was sitting at the table next to mine. He was haranguing his table, ranting that we all had to be careful as Islam was going to take over Europe. He had obviously bought into the new theory of the clash of civilizations. The entire table listened without reacting, everyone staring at their plate. This patient turned out to live in the same building in Lausanne as my friend Nabil. I remembered catching sight of him in the lobby during one of my visits a few years ago. Although they do not chat to each other, they exchange greetings. Nabil is Muslim, his neighbour is Jewish.

There was also a modest lady from Renens, a working-class suburb of Lausanne. In her sixties, she had always lived in the same neighbourhood. She described how it had changed over the years, with lots of foreigners moving in. She was sweet, softly-spoken and did not complain, so I didn't know how she really felt about this. But I got the impression that it disturbed her.

Returning to Fernand, I found out that his daughter had been beaten up by a group of young people in Monthey, for obscure reasons. Her swollen face had been in the headlines. I remember seeing this picture on the front page of the daily Le Matin. This affair had attracted a great deal of publicity. The young offenders turned out to be foreigners. The case and media coverage had stirred up hatred against foreigners, a sensitive issue in Switzerland at that time (and even more topical nowadays due to the arrival of refugees). When I asked Fernand about this, he just said, "That will teach her not to trust everyone". I understand that this girl had a good heart and often gave young people a place to stay.

This move to the "common area" allowed me to meet a wide range of people from all walks of life. It was a microcosm that exposed the realities of this multifaceted society. It led me to rediscover, or even discover, the country of my birth and how it had changed for better and for worse, in particular with regard to the problems linked to immigration, in the thirty years since I had left it.

I discovered a changed country. I had been made aware of these changes by the media and discussions with my family and friends, but now I was confronted with them for real. At the end of the day we were no different from the rest of Europe. My conception of the Swiss exception, a country different from the others, floundered.

The opportunity to rediscover my country from the inside turned out to be one of the most interesting and positive aspects of my illness.

PRIVILEGED

And then there were the other patients: those who had been devastated by strokes that had left them practically unable to communicate.

One man used to wander the corridor; unable to speak he would wail instead. Often he would roar, which startled Wanda. He must have been in his late forties. The occupational therapists, using yes-no questions (he nodded to answer) managed to guess his former job: electrician. This was a sad case as it seemed unlikely that he would recover any time soon, if at all.

I befriended an elderly well-to-do gentleman from Geneva and his wife. He too had suffered a stroke that had left him unable to speak. But he was calm and smiling, shaking his head to show he understood. The couple had come here specifically for Bogousslavsky. They had high hopes of him, but I feared that he would not be able to do much to help.

Another patient, a peaky-looking old lady was assigned to my table for meals. She could not speak either. Despite this and the fact that her neck was in a support, she smiled all the time.

There were other relatively less serious cases of partial paralysis. But all seemed chronic and impossible to cure. The most that could be done was to stabilize their condition.

One woman had multiple sclerosis. She was an acquaintance of Laurence Jacquet, a friend of the family. She had to be at the clinic for a check-up and took the opportunity to come and see me. She was walking with a stick but, according to Laurence, she was in a stable, positive phase. She encouraged me, which is remarkable, considering that her condition was much more serious than mine. Multiple sclerosis bears similarities to Guillain Barré: both are autoimmune diseases and attack myelin. But multiple sclerosis attacks the central nervous system, not the peripheral. It is a much more vicious disease as it is chronic and can be accompanied by a lot of pain.

Seeing all these people, I felt almost privileged as at least there was a chance that I would heal. My condition was almost benign in comparison. Moreover, I was making progress and owed it to myself to be positive. The path was long, but I would get there.

A BRIEF HISTORY OF VALMONT

I had been in Valmont for more than three months. "I'm becoming part of the furniture," I told myself. By this time I could move much more independently. I could transfer from my bed to the wheelchair and get around quickly.

I began to take an interest in the history of Valmont. This monumental Art Nouveau clinic was inaugurated in 1905. Initially it was reserved for the wealthy and only became more open later on. A multitude of celebrities have been treated here including Vladimir Nabokov, Georges Simenon, Julien Green, Richard Attenborough, Charlie Chaplin, Ingrid Bergman, Coco Chanel, Grace Jones and Placido Domingo, to name just a few. King Albert of Belgium, Princess Soraya of Iran and President Mobutu have also received treatment here. During my stay, a fellow patient told me that she had spotted Maurice Béjart, the famous choreographer, quietly coming out of the pool, outside normal hours.[4]

One of the most prominent personalities to stay here was probably the Austrian poet and writer Rainer Maria Rilke who was treated here three times in the 1920s suffering from incurable leukaemia. He died here in December 1926 at the age of 51. I discovered that Rilke had occupied room 323 during his second stay, a room that was later transformed into the bathroom I was now using. Even though I was not very familiar with this poet, this information gave me a strange feeling and made me want to learn more about him. I found out that he spent the last years of his life in Valais, Switzerland and that he also wrote in French. I started reading and appreciating his poems.

First I had rediscovered my country, and now thanks to Valmont, I was exploring the fascinating history of this region. This, in combination with my homecoming, the closeness of my family, my childhood and youth friends, especially my almost one hundred-year-old father, gave me an incredible feeling of richness. I had rediscovered my roots.

The wanderer returned. This was one of the good sides of my Guillain Barré.

NABIL

"Paul, Nabil has just had a heart attack." It was Christina, my friend Nabil's wife on the phone. "He is in the hospital in Lausanne". She was panicked. "He is crazy, he had that pain in his chest but insisted on driving himself to the hospital rather than wait for an ambulance."

Fortunately, things were less serious than expected and Nabil did not need a coronary artery bypass as feared. He got off with angioplasty, i.e. having a stent (a thin catheter topped with a small balloon) inserted in the narrowed artery. The hospital kept him in for a few days and prescribed a fortnight of rest for him. I called him: "Nabil, why don't you come to Valmont? They treat heart patients here."

So, my old friend Nabil joined me in Valmont for his compulsory rest: two old study mates in a rehabilitation clinic. We had to laugh, saying: "We used to go to the pub but now, at our age, we hang out at the hospital".

We shared our meals at his table, near the window. By now I was walking tentatively, using a stick. At the end of the meal he would pull me up from behind by my belt (my legs were still very weak), give me my walking stick and we would go for a little stroll around the building.

Nabil was an impossible patient. He could not survive without his mobile and always had it with him ready to answer calls; he worked for a bank and wanted to keep up with what was happening. After a few attempts the staff gave up trying to confiscate it, concluding that it would do him more harm than good. He also took his car, a big Mercedes, even though he was not allowed to drive until he was better. One evening, we went to Villeneuve to eat perch fillets, accompanied by two North African nursing assistants whom Nabil had invited. I do not know what he was thinking, but the sight of two middle-aged patients, one of whom could hardly walk, in the company of these young ladies must have been quite comical. Once again we were the mischievous boys we had been at university.

FALLINGS

I was walking again. By then it was late April and I had been ill for five months. I needed a walking frame in the beginning but I soon progressed to a walking stick. Although my legs were still very weak, they were strong enough to support me. I became obsessed with the fear of falling.

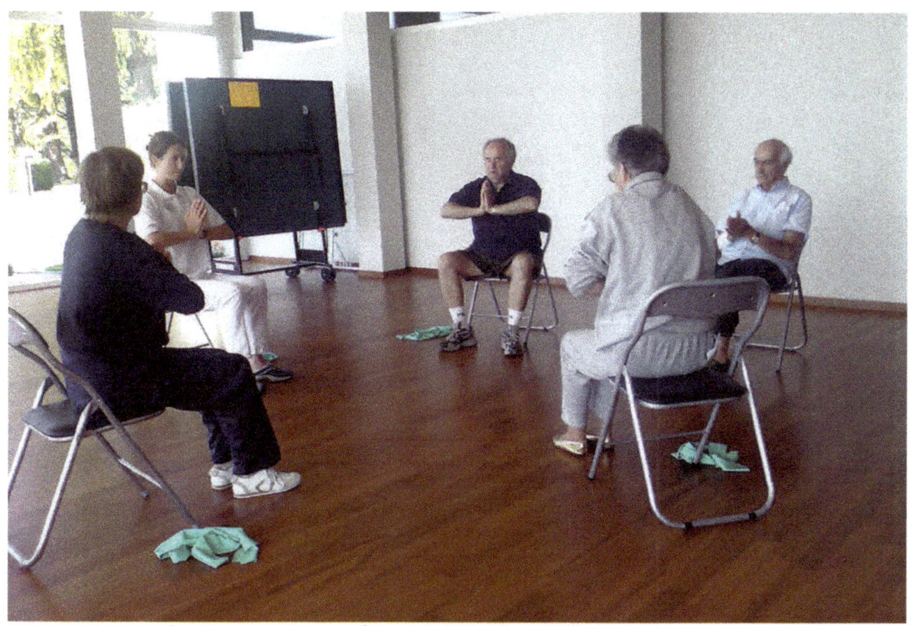

Heart patient meditation exercise, my friend Nabil in the middle

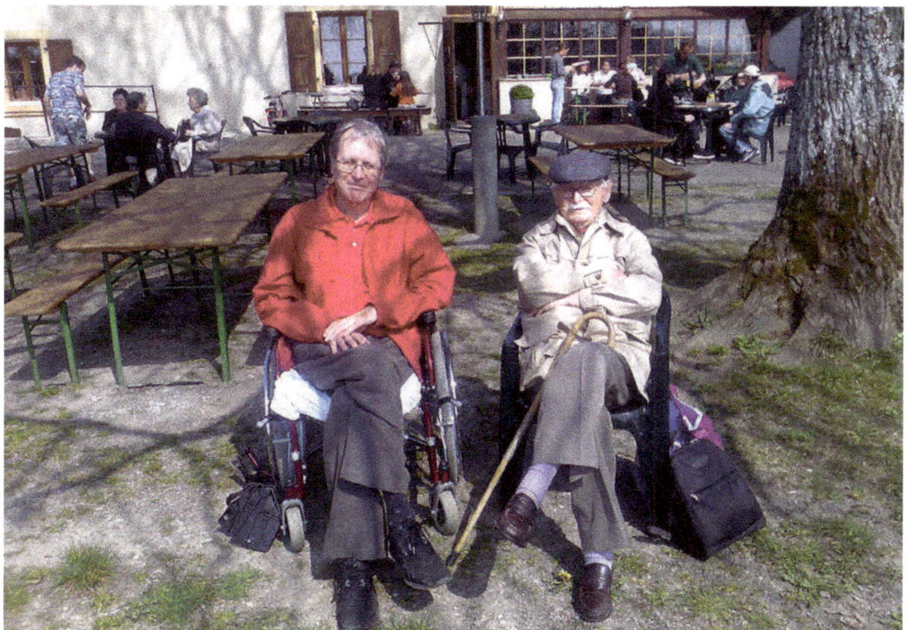

Together with my 99 year old father Emilio who would say: "you are going up, I am go down"

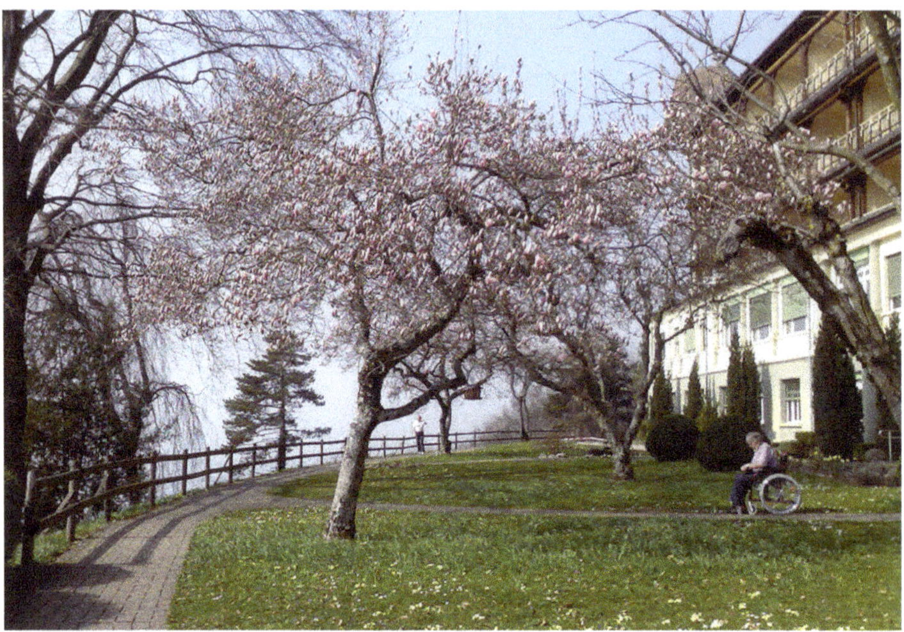

Cherry blossoms

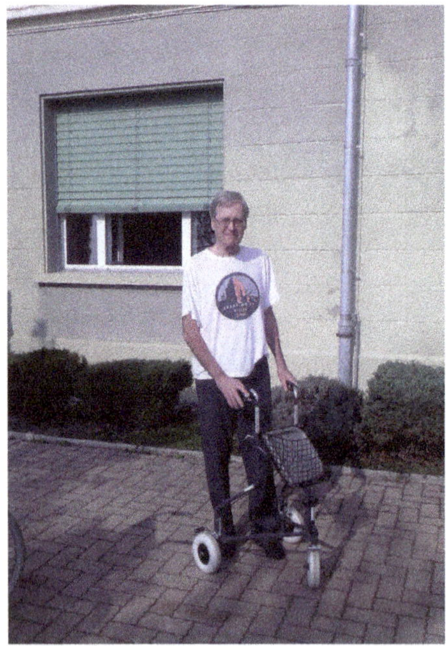

Walking frame

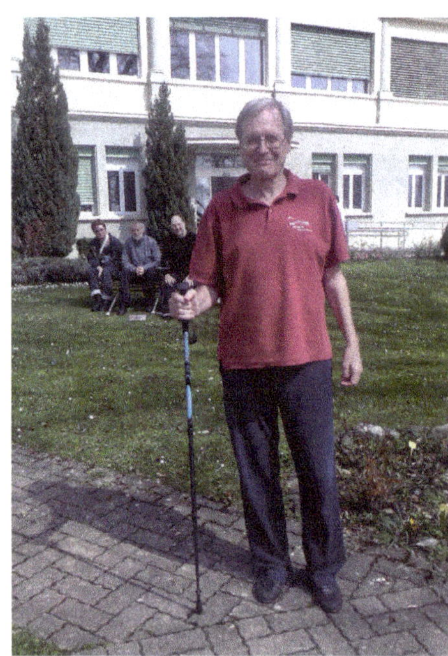

Walking stick

My first fall was when I was undressing to go to bed. I stood on one leg to remove my trousers and crashed to the floor, unable to break my fall. My legs just gave way under me. Fortunately, I was not hurt but I could not get up. I had to call for the nurse to heave me onto the bed. The next day at my occupational therapy session, Catherine, my therapist, commented: "Ah, you fell last night, you must be careful".

The same thing happened to Mrs Wilke, my partner in misfortune, who was also starting to use the walking frame. All the therapists knew: "Mrs Wilke fell and hurt herself, she will need at least two weeks to recover".

I fell three times during my weekend outings but did not tell anyone. The first time was in Villeneuve during an outing with my father, when my legs gave way without warning. Maybe I shouldn't have had that glass of wine with my meal. I was helped back on my feet by one of my companions. The second time was during my second visit to Le Trétien, when I fell on the terrace steps. Once more my legs had simply given up on me. I lay on the ground sobbing. Wanda didn't know what to do but finally I managed to get up with her help, once more uninjured. The third time was at my father's, when I was trying to get into bed. I fell trying to move an armchair. This time I hurt my knee but the pain was bearable. I continued my exercises as if nothing had happened. These falls undermined my spirits. They meant a delay in my recovery and I felt ashamed whenever I had to admit to them.

Looking back I find this attitude rather weird. Why be ashamed? But I had adopted a combative attitude, I struggled to recover and did not accept defeat. For me a fall was like a blow below the belt to sabotage my recovery.

THE LAST TWO MONTHS - SPRING

By April, spring was well underway. In-between my occupational therapy and physiotherapy sessions I spent a lot of time enjoying the sun in the garden. I saw the first daffodils and the cherry tree was in bloom. I photographed everything. The most able-bodied patients were also there, sitting on a bench, walking slowly with a walking frame or being pushed around in a wheelchair. I appreciated the calm and serenity. The noise of the motorway was much less audible from the garden than from my balcony.

By now I could also get on the balcony by myself, first by manoeuvring my wheelchair over the threshold, later by walking carefully. Finally, I was able to enjoy the view of the lake and the Alps to the south, the Rhone plain with the Dents du Midi to the east and the Jura range to the west. The unobstructed view made me forget the hum of the motorway traffic below. Around mid-May, a series of thunderstorms confined us inside. The view from the balcony was phantasmagorical, with veiled sunsets in the clouds, mornings with dense fog and endless, almost tropical rainfall.

In April my employer's Human Resources department in Breda contacted me about my repatriation to the Netherlands. The insurance company had not forgotten me. They wanted me to come home. The nervous little French doctor came to see me: "They are asking me when you will be able to leave. How do I know? I cannot predict how you will be in two or three weeks." It was as if he was asking me to decide. I listened and said nothing. One or two weeks elapsed without any news. Finally, Dr. Bogousslavski made the decision. By this time, it was early May and on one of his routine visits he said: "They are asking us when you can return to the Netherlands. They want you to come home. I told them that, given your progress, you should be able to leave within three weeks, towards the end of May."

It was difficult to decide upon a date in cases like mine. It was the same with Christiane Wilke: her insurance company was putting a lot of pressure on her to leave the rehabilitation centre, even though she was not really ready. She could hardly walk and her hands were still paralysed. She was hit harder than me. To her relief the doctors managed to get her an extra three weeks.

By this time I had an excellent relationship with Dr. Bogousslavsky and he appreciated my progress. Shortly before my departure he asked me if I wanted to serve as a guinea pig for a briefing on Guillain-Barré for Valmont employees. I gladly agreed, telling myself it was for a good cause. The session lasted about twenty minutes. The entire medical staff, around twenty people, attended. Bogousslavsky made me do some exercises, lift my arms, bend my legs, etc. Folding my legs was still painful as I had fallen the previous weekend at my father's house. My knee was swollen but I did not mention this as I did not want to delay my recovery. No one noticed anything and everything went well.

At our final meeting before I left, the neurologist reiterated his satisfaction regarding my progress: "I am really pleasantly surprised, you have made excellent progress". To my question of whether there was any chance of relapse, he replied: "No, you would be really unlucky if it happened again". When I expressed my worries about my libido and sexual activity he reassured me by saying: "Don't worry, it will come back".

I arrived back in the Netherlands on Sunday, June 3. A nursing assistant accompanied me on the flight from Geneva. My friend Pete Purnell was waiting for me at the airport to take me home.

I had spent 5 months of my life in Valmont.

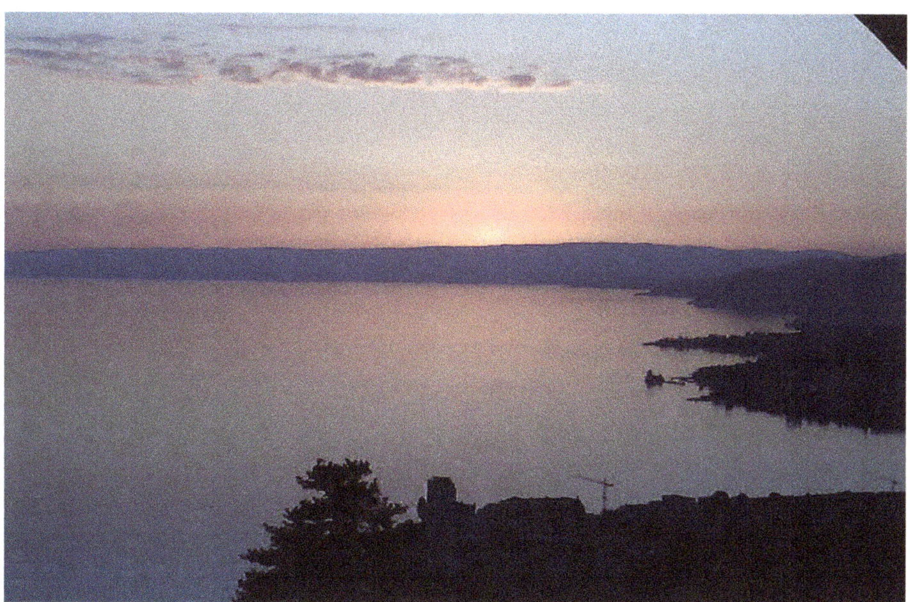

Sunset from my balcony, Lake Geneva and Jura mountains in the background

CHAPTER FOUR

AMSTERDAM

Summer is coming. But it only comes to those who know how to wait, as quiet and open as if they had eternity ahead of them.
- Rainer Maria Rilke

"We will continue to treat you for as long as there is progress. But once that stops, we will stop too. I think you can understand that." These were the words of my neurologist at the Rehabilitation Centre in Amsterdam (RCA) [5] during our introductory interview. A relatively young woman in her late thirties, she was serious, like all the other neurologists I had dealt with. She was rational, down to earth and did not mince her words. The Dutch have a word for this attitude: "nuchter". It is one of the chief characteristics of this country, which owes so much to Calvinism.

I could sense neither encouragement nor discouragement in her words. At least she did not advise me to move to a house with no stairs. She made it clear that the ball was now in my court. I was prescribed physiotherapy sessions three days a week, plus occupational therapy. The rehabilitation centre was two kilometres away from my house and I walked there, using the walking stick I had been given in Valmont. It took me about half an hour.

Due to various problems, my treatment was delayed by almost a month, and did not start until early July. In the meantime, a young, likeable practitioner came to give me physiotherapy at home, mainly consisting of accompanied one-hour walks around my neighbourhood two or three times a week.

Climbing up and down the steep stairs at home was good exercise and I handled it relatively well, moving slowly and carefully, pulling myself up on the bannister. My friend René Lesson installed a guardrail along the three steps leading to the garden. For the rest, it was not difficult to adapt to living at home again. Wanda bought a chair with armrests for the dining table so that I could push myself up, and social services provided us with a bath board to make bathing easier. But no other changes were required.

RCA

Eric [1], my regular physiotherapist was a lanky fellow with curly brown hair and a serious expression, somewhere in his thirties. He had a very similar attitude and approach to Grégoire, my physiotherapist at Valmont. Like Grégoire, he was a fan of 100% physiotherapy, with no frills. Instead, he pushed me to my limits. In September, Eric told me to cycle to the centre instead of walking. This was a huge challenge. Although my legs were a little bit stronger, there was no way I could cycle up a slope. It's a good job that Amsterdam is almost flat! However, I was worried about the small arched bridge on my route and got off the bike midway in case I slid backwards. There was also a difficult junction at Overtoom/ Nassaukade that hardly gave cyclists any time to cross the road. I could barely manage as I didn't have the strength to pedal fast, but somehow I did it. The first time was quite stressful but I soon got used to it. I even made the occasional detour through Vondelpark. Without Eric nudging me I would never have dared to cycle again so soon.

LE TRÉTIEN

At the end of July, we drove to Switzerland to spend the summer at our chalet in Le Trétien with Wanda and her mother Jadwiga – known as Baba to close friends – who had arrived from Warsaw. The calm and serenity of the mountains did us good. I practiced walking, using my stick. Every other day I would go to buy bread from Madame Lina, who ran the little grocery store in the upper part of the village. The steep slope was good exercise for me. Occasionally the tiny shop was closed, so I would ring the bell and Madame Lina, who lived above the shop, would hobble down the stairs on her swollen legs. She must have been in her eighties. Although the store had not made a profit for a long time, she was determined to keep it going; it was her life. We used to swap our experiences about walking. I would tell her how I had managed to climb the slope without stopping, she would congratulate me and tell me about her sore leg.

My cousin from Australia, Christian, and his wife Pamela, visited us at Le Trétien, bringing my father, Emilio, with them. Wanda took a picture of Emilio with Minouche, our neighbour's cat, sitting on his lap. This photo will illustrate the back cover of my father's memoirs.

On August 17, we celebrated Wanda's birthday. We rented the old school hall and invited Polish, Irish and other friends from all over Europe. Our friends from the village, Mado and Christian, the Pittinos, Pierre André and Danielle, Dédé and many others also joined us, and even our old neighbour, Lucien, dropped in. My family from Lausanne came and so, of course, did my father. He was thrilled when we took a photo of him surrounded by women. Dear Don Emilio was a charmer until the end. We danced until late in the evening, and even I made a few tentative steps on the dance floor. It was a fantastic party which will be remembered in the valley for a long time to come. Our Polish guests definitely made an impression. I felt happy, as if normal life had finally resumed.

It was around that time that I started keeping a diary.

Excerpt from my diary: *"September 7, 2007: back to Le Trétien for a few days. Today walked up to Finhaut. First time this year (and since the Guillain). Things are getting better little by little. Patience, patience. Everything will work out. I am always in good spirits."*

ELTON JOHN
On September 8, Elton John gave an open-air concert in Vevey, in the main market square. This unique event fell on my birthday and in my birthplace. Although I was not a real fan, I didn't want to miss it. Time for a brief visit to Switzerland! By then I had just started walking without a stick.

The show was disappointing, mainly because of the acoustics. The sound bounced off the nearby buildings, creating interference and making the music virtually inaudible, especially for those standing at the back, like us.

Elton did not look very inspired. He just worked through the numbers in a humdrum fashion, without any feeling or interaction with the audience. The 2 hour concert seemed to go on forever as I stood there shifting my weight from one leg to the other.

At the end of the concert, around 10 pm, I stumbled and fell. Everyone around me thought I was drunk and made comments to that effect. Luckily, Wanda was there to help me back on my feet but I was exhausted by standing for so long.

The next day, I read in the local press that the organizers of the concert were also disappointed, but for other reasons. They had planned a supper for Elton John at the end of the concert and had reserved a room for him at Hotel des Trois Couronnes, an extremely chic hotel with breath-taking views of the lake. But Elton had other plans: he went home straight after the show, taking off in a helicopter to Geneva and from there to London.

WELCOME TO THE REAL WORLD
Back in Amsterdam, I resumed my physiotherapy sessions at the rehabilitation centre. I was now walking without the stick. This was a significant step, as it signified my "return" to the real world. Without my walking stick, I blended into the crowd, no longer recognizable as an invalid. People stopped making extra allowances for me.

One Saturday I went on my own to the city centre, a twenty-minute walk from our house. I crossed Munt square, which was buzzing with people. Suddenly I stumbled, fell to the ground and couldn't get up. There I was in the middle of a pedestrian crossing, kneeling on the ground, looking around me, while everyone passed me by without so much as a glance. As in Vevey, people must have thought that I was an alcoholic. I stayed there, gesturing, trying but failing to get up for what seemed like an eternity (it was probably only thirty seconds) before finally a Spanish tourist, all smiles, came running towards me and helped me back on my feet.

Another great moment came on September 21, when at the insistence of my physiotherapist, I managed to get up by myself for the first time. This was an enormous step and I wrote in my diary: *"Today I managed to get up on my own. A BIG MILESTONE. Now I am really beginning to believe it: I will get back to 100% I WANT IT "*.

It was around that time I started cycling, following the physiotherapist's encouragments.

I also started driving. How liberating to be able to drive a car! It felt as if the world belonged to me again, as if I had wings, as if I had returned to normality.

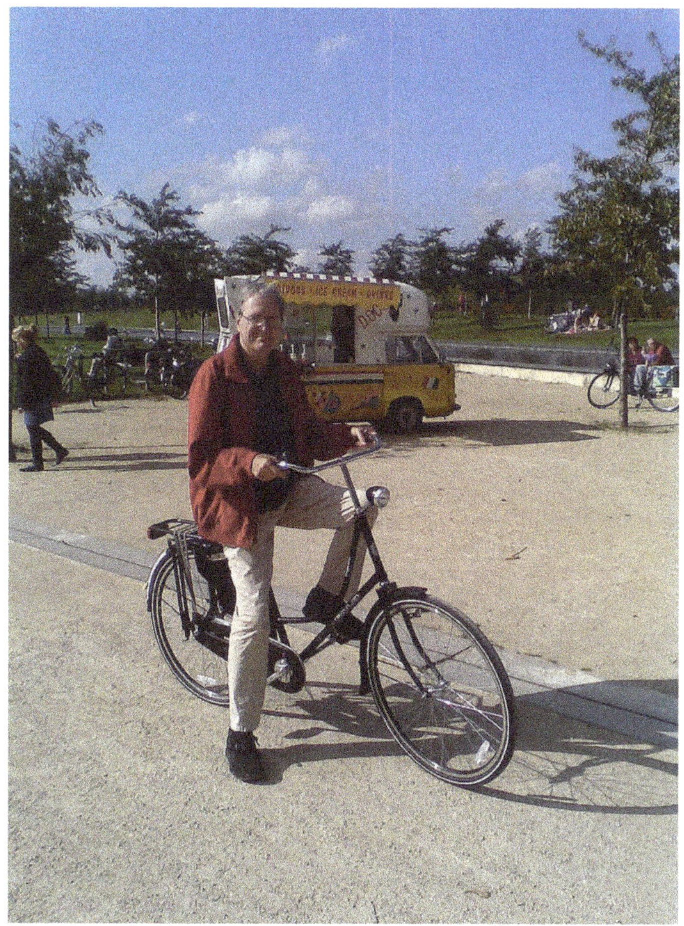

First ride on the bicycle   © Wanda Michalak

On September 26, I drove on my own to Rotterdam to see the company doctor Kees van Rooy. After a brief consultation, he said I could go back to work on November 5. He stated two reasons: I should be physically fit enough to return to work by then and, more urgently, he explained that after one year of incapacity for work (I had been off work since late November 2006), my health insurance coverage would plummet. This was a convincing reason to return to work. The doctor suggested that I work just three days a week for the first three months to ease my way back in. This seemed like a reasonable proposal.

EXCERPTS FROM MY DIARY
September 26, 2007:
"Today interview with the company doctor. Proposal to resume work as from November 5. This sounds good to me.

A little depressed today: a classic but still fundamental question: what is life for?

I had the rare opportunity to think and reflect about it for almost a year. But what is the outcome? Not much frankly.

Everything seems trivial to me. Work especially. Budget problem? Trifling. But the rest too. To read, OK, but it is just a way of evading the issue. I read very little this year. And yet I had plenty of time. Well, at first there were concentration problems. But only the first month. After that there was no excuse. Watch movies? OK, but it is really a way out. Listen to music? Always nice. I do it very often. I am busy transferring all my music to I-Tunes. But that also gets tiresome. There are too many and I lose control.

Take care of the gallery? [6] *OK, that is good. But it's not really my thing. I can't do much besides helping with the administration. But at least, it occupies me a little.*

In fact, the only thing that really interests me right now is my fight to get better. I like physiotherapy but don't get enough. I like cycling, weather permitting.

I like being physically active. I like my body. Getting back to 100% is a beautiful goal. Everything else seems trivial to me right now."

Sunday, November 4, 2007:
"I am on "duty" in the gallery. Beautiful exhibition at the moment: Renan Cepeda – "Light painting". Sold a few pieces – only a pity there are not more visitors.

But those who come enjoy it a lot. To date, sold 8 catalogues (+ 5 during the preview).
I feel much better these days. The past few weeks I have been walking a little faster. I still have difficulty climbing stairs and standing up. But this is also progressing slowly.

I stopped going to the revalidation centre (RCA) two weeks ago. I now go to the Splash fitness centre three times a week for strengthening exercises under the supervision of a physiotherapist. Only a one-minute walk from my house, very convenient. The sessions last an hour and after two weeks I can see progress, especially in my legs. I should have gone there earlier.

I was very active last week. I did a lot of cycling. I went twice to the cinema on my own. Went to a ballet with Wanda. Went to see a concert of the Dutch group "De Kift" at the Melkweg with René. Then went to my friend Gerrit's 60th birthday party (took a taxi). Everything went well. I feel like I am getting back to life and have more lust for life...

...Next week I resume work. I will assist Sharon Meachen in Paris. I start part time. I have mixed feelings about returning to work. On the one hand, I would have liked to wait until the end of the year and enjoy some of my free time now that I have almost recovered and have regained my independence. On the other hand, I think it is good to go back to real life. I hope it will accelerate my total recovery. Life is beautiful, you have to enjoy every moment".

DRIVING LICENCE
At the end of October, during my final interview with the revalidation centre in Amsterdam, the neurologist, whom I had met only once before during my admission, was shocked when I told her that I was driving again: "That's not possible. Do not do that. If anything happens you will not be covered by insurance". I had been driving for at least two months. I had even driven on my own to Brussels, 200 km from Amsterdam, to undergo treatment for a non-malignant skin cancer on my face. I had also driven in Switzerland. She strongly recommended that I stay away from the steering wheel. This was a setback, as being back behind the wheel had been so liberating. I had not realized that I should have been more careful. When I explained that I was going back to work and would probably need to drive, she sent me for a medical examination to test

whether I was fit to do so.

I passed the test successfully one month later. It consisted of driving around a block, parking manoeuvres and braking at top speed on a straight line. They measured the pressure of my foot on the brake pedal using a device placed under it. The examiner, a very nice doctor, asked me to press my foot down as hard as I could; first my left foot then the right. She concluded that I had enough strength, although the measured force of the right foot was just below the required minimum. She decided that the device was poorly calibrated and passed me. I was licensed for a period of five years. Life was back to normal.

5 years later, my licence was renewed automatically, without my having to undergo another examination.

SPLASH

I was at Splash, the gym, where I had been going since mid-November for my muscle-development exercises. That day I was doing weight lifting to strengthen my arms. This was sorely needed as I could hardly lift 15 kilos. Right next to me, a hefty guy was lying on his back, doing bench presses with a weight of 150 kilos. He did five lifts in a row, breathing heavily, the sweat dripping from his face. There I was with my miserable 15 kilos, feeling ridiculous in comparison. My physiotherapist told me that the athlete was Swiss, like me: what a coincidence. He turned out to be from Upper Valais and had been living in Amsterdam for some time. As he didn't speak French and I don't understand his dialect – Upper Valaisan is incomprehensible even for other Swiss-Germans – we communicated in Dutch. He was keen on kickboxing – apparently Amsterdam was a well-known centre for this Asian martial sport – and regularly trained at Splash. He was a real Swiss with gnarled arms and when I learnt of his nationality I had to laugh and exclaimed: "Well, we really have the two extremes of Swiss athletes: 15 kilos against 150!" He smiled as he went about his exercises.

CHAPTER FIVE

NEW LIFE

"We look like two old cripples, look what the company has done to us," said my colleague Tom Mangold, grinning as we both slowly climbed the steps of this tall building, which was undergoing renovation in Paris La Défense.

I had gone back to work for three days a week. My task was to assist my New Zealand colleague Sharon Meachen, who was managing a major office development project in Paris. I was reunited with my old friend, colleague and mentor Tom Mangold, who was retired but had been rehired to share his experience as a consultant. That morning he was showing me around the building site that covered three floors of the building. Tom had Parkinson's disease: although he could not write because of his tremors, he could manage on the computer. He was in his sixties and this job was keeping him going. But there we were, struggling to climb the steps, clinging to the bannister, like two old men. You had to see the funny side of the situation. Tom's remark made us laugh so much we had to stop for a break. He continued: "We should warn the new generation of what they can expect if they take on this crazy job". This set us off again.

I travelled to Paris every week on Thalys, the high-speed train. It was a comfortable trip lasting about four hours (the Dutch section was not yet at high speed). During the first trip I spilled my coffee on my neighbour's papers while trying to take the cup from the steward with my right hand. Some arm movements can cause tremors in my hands, an uncontrollable nervous reaction. Luckily my neighbour didn't seem too annoyed. Maybe he had noticed that I was slightly handicapped. From that day on I always grabbed objects with both hands. I usually spent two nights in Paris, in a hotel in La Défense to the west of the city, very near the construction site.

"Do not travel by metro, take a taxi instead", were Sharon's first words when we met, surprising me by speaking French. Sharon was worried about me as she knew about my situation and didn't want the trip to wear me out. It felt strange to be back at work. Sharon introduced me to the various members of the project team. Everything was fast, everyone was busy. It was like landing in a beehive: there were meetings going on and people were rushing here and there. It made me dizzy. For months I had been living at a slower pace in relative tranquillity, only occupied with myself. But now I was back in the world of work. Sharon had very little time for me, as she was busy answering the phone and instructing her team. She briefly explained how I could assist her. She proposed I take care of a "satellite" project, the construction of a small office for the representatives of lubes sales in Saint-Denis, on the outskirts of Paris, as she did not have time for this project. She gave me the file, a few explanations and the rest was up to me.

During my third visit to Paris, I discovered that there would be a taxi strike for the next two days. This was not usual. France is well known for its strikes, but they generally affect the public sector. Strikes in the private sector are rare, but plans had just been announced to liberalize the taxi system. This was before Uber but already the market was beginning to change. I found myself forced to use the metro, a hellish experience. I had never realised that the corridors were so long, that there were so many stairs and that there were not escalators everywhere. Having to carry my suitcase around made matters even worse. When I was leaving Paris I somehow managed to get from La Défense to Gare du Nord, changing at Les Halles, in the heart of the city. When I finally sat down in my reserved seat in the train I heaved a sigh of relief.

After a few weeks I was sick of spending the evenings alone in my hotel room in La Défense far from all the action. One late afternoon, after work, I plucked up my courage and took the metro into town. It was not complicated as it's a direct line with no changes (line 1). I got off at Charles de Gaulle-Étoile at the foot of the Arc de Triomphe and walked to Avenue des Champs-Elysées. After a few metres, I stumbled on a cobblestone and fell on the sidewalk. A passer-by immediately rushed to help me. "I am fine, don't worry, thank you," I said, managing to get up on my own. Although that fall did not discourage me too much, I cut my walk short and returned to the hotel.

Munt square in Amsterdam, the Market square in Vevey and now the Champs-Élysées: I sure picked my places to fall over.

EMILIO'S 100th BIRTHDAY

On February 8, 2008, we celebrated Emilio's 100th birthday at the Château de La Tour-de-Peilz, at Lake Geneva. The whole family was there, including my German Swiss relatives. My cousins Richard and Christian from Australia were there too. Wanda was with me, Baba had come from Warsaw and Sebastian from Amsterdam. There were about sixty guests in total. It was wonderful. My brother Raymond had organized everything. I was the master of ceremonies, my nephew Robin made a beautiful speech. After the meal, everyone gathered in the garden for a group photo. The weather was fine, wind still, and the low February sun shone brightly, blinding us with its reflections on the lake. It was impossible to adequately appreciate this great blue, immobile liquid mass. It was like a sea of mercury surrounded on the horizon by the Jura mountains. Everyone was enjoying themselves and Emilio was in seventh heaven. He was asked to sign his memoirs, which we had published and reissued for the occasion (70 copies, one for everyone present). It was a great success and I am happy that I was able to contribute to it.

My father died five months later, in July 2008, without suffering, following a stroke. He was lucid and dignified until the end. I am grateful to fate for allowing me to be with him so often during this final phase of his life and to share many weekends with him. This was one of the positive aspects of my illness.

KILL THE DEMON?

In April 2008, I went to N'Djamena, Chad, for the final administrative closure of the office building project (work had been completed more than a year earlier) and to verify that all documents were complete and in good order so that an audit could be held five months later in September.

Audits were not to be taken lightly. Following a corruption scandal in the Italian subsidiary in the 1980s, our company was obsessed with them. If mistakes were made, one could expect a severe reprimand or even demotion. Farsi and Amos, two former members of the project team, were there to assist me in that task.

Two months earlier, in February 2008, an attempted coup had seriously undermined the country. A rebel offensive, launched on N'Djamena against President Idriss Déby Ito's regime, had nearly achieved its goal. The rebels had moved swiftly on the capital from the east of the country but the president stayed in his palace, refusing to leave the country. The army remained faithful and the insurrection was put down after two days of fighting. This was partly thanks to the crucial role played by the French air force which has a base in the country. People shut themselves up in their homes and foreign residents were evacuated. There were hundreds of casualties, especially in the ranks of the insurgents, and looting was rife. This was the second takeover attempt within two years.

My colleague Patrick Hervier told me that when entering the city, one of the rebel columns as it run past the company's headquarters, which had been evacuated, fired shots in the air to intimidate the civilians. One of the bullets got lodged in the "chiller", the water cooling unit, located on the roof of the building, shutting down the air conditioning.

Two months later, the situation had completely normalised, everyone had returned to the country and the company was allowing visitors like me to return. Even the "chiller" had been repaired.

I was there for a week. I stayed in Tréguer, the "staff house" which is located near our offices on the Avenue de Bordeaux, a beaten-earth road. This was where I had stayed during the project. Except for a few extra cracks Tréguer hadn't changed. The staff were the same and Mr Mohammed was still in charge. Meals were still served in the small refectory on the ground floor. The menu had not changed either; still rice with either meat or chicken. We nicknamed the legendary chicken legs the "bicycle" as they consisted of skin and bone with a tiny bit of flesh in-between. I had eaten a great deal of chicken in Africa.

Mr Mohammed, smiling, asked me: "Do you know Chadian music?" I looked at him questioningly, he continued: "It is the sound of machine guns". The recent rebellion attempt was still in everyone's mind.

Sunday, April 20, 2008, excerpt from my diary

"Just arrived at N'Djamena. First visit since my illness. Last time I was here was September 2006! Same reception, same driver, even Tréguer (with some more cracks), same road (with detours because of repairs at the Carnivore restaurant). At first sight nothing had fundamentally changed. It was as if I was there yesterday, except that I had trouble climbing the stairs and into the minibus. This was when I noticed that I had changed.

Same nice people. They all recognized me and were apparently happy to see me. I saw my colleague Heather at the airport. She was really happy to see me in good health.

It is 11 pm European time, 10 pm local time. I am in room 104. We will see how things go tomorrow. One thing is certain: I am really happy to be here. It is important to return to the places where I was before my illness, especially here, where I spent a significant part of my life. I feel it is part of the therapy (the ultimate therapy would be to go back to Lagos, but we are not there yet)."

I used to walk the 200 metres between Tréguer and the offices, even though company safety procedures advised us to go by car. But as our security officer, who was French, said: "There is really not a bandit hiding behind every tree". The local population was very friendly and the children were always happy to see us. I remember that my colleague Nora brought them sweets every time she came. A few goats grazed on the scant blades of grass protruding from the dust at the edge of the road. The sun beat down. It must have been around 38–40 degrees but at least you don't sweat too much in such an arid climate.

As I approached the offices, I heard the hiss of the "chiller", the famous air conditioning cooling unit on the roof of the building. It was working better than ever as there was enough power. And there, suddenly, something was triggered in my mind: that noise stirred the memory of the generators and all the problems they had caused. The constant, shrill hissing of the chiller began to obsess me and pierce my skull.

Everything came flooding back: that hellish night two years ago, alone in my room in Tréguer, when I had started to panic. My fears that an unavoidable generator failure would deprive the offices of power and air conditioning. The entire film replayed in my memory.

I had been a fool for thinking that this problem was inescapable and insoluble. Could this have been the cause of all my troubles? Could this have been the root of the evil?

The demon! It was the demon! The demon of stress! That's what was to blame for everything!

All of a sudden, everything became clear to me: the demon of stress had taken hold of me in that place. He had subtly bewitched me and decided to attack me the following year, on Mount Cameroon, disguising himself as a chicken.

The demon had been identified. The reason I had returned was to face him, unmask him and try to banish him.

I was here to KILL THE DEMON.

Sunday, April 27, excerpt from my diary

"I am here to kill the demon. Funny impression after all. Is it possible that my illness has its roots in this place? Just hearing the shrill hissing of the chiller on the roof of the building brings back terrible memories of the project, when we feared that the generators could fail at any time, with no possibility of replacement in the immediate future. That terrible period when I went round in circles all night in my room in Tréguer, practically climbing the walls. It was in December 2005, a year before my attack of Guillain-Barré. The extreme stress may have been the cause of this immune deficiency."

I extended my stay in Chad by four days. We needed more time to put all the documentation in order and be ready for the September audit. Farsi and Amos' assistance was crucial. I needed the time this extension gave me to confront the demon as I was not sure I could eradicate it completely in one go.

"Tonight, a fit of the blues. I feel I do not make much progress with my legs. It seems to be stagnating. I am here to kill the demon. The demon will not survive". (excerpt from my diary)

Perhaps I should have copied the rebels and shot the chiller to silence it? After all, it was definitely connected to the roots of my illness. But it would only be repaired.

Finally, I had to accept that I could not banish the demon yet. Identifying him, however, was a major step in the right direction. I was no longer fighting ghosts. Now that I knew what I was dealing with, I could try to keep it under control. This gave me energy and renewed my determination to continue my fight. I left N'Djamena with plenty of optimism in my luggage.

The Chadian project was audited in September 2008 as planned. The verdict was "satisfactory", a very positive outcome for our company. That was a victory for me as some malicious tongues had anticipated a failure. That result lifted my spirits: another new step in the right direction! The demon was being brought under control. I would no longer submit to its dominion.

A NEW LIFE

In spring 2008 I went back to work full time. In May I was sent to Luanda, Angola, to oversee the final phase of a construction project for Torres Atlântico, a major real estate complex in the heart of the city. I was replacing my colleague George Dyche, who had been sent to another mission which had been scheduled ages ago and could not wait any longer.

My mission in Angola was supposed to last 4 months, but I ended up staying there for 18 months. Because of my disability I was given preferential treatment and allowed to stay in an apartment adjacent to our temporary office just a stone's throw from the construction site.

Torres Atlântico comprised two towers: a commercial tower with 19 floors of offices and a residential tower with 15 floors of flats. The towers were separated by a leisure area with a swimming pool and fitness area. The complex was owned by three oil companies: Esso, BP and Sonangol, the latter being an Angolan state-owned company. The total budget for the operation was in the region of 360 million dollars. A Portuguese property developer was in charge of construction, which started in 2005.

As an "operator", Esso was in charge of monitoring construction and coordination with the developer. In other words, we represented the other two co-owners and were in charge of budget control, quality and planning. We also established the compulsory safety standards for the developer and his construction company.

This was a prestigious project for the Angolan government: located on a prominent site on the coast, it was a symbol of the country's rebirth. [7] Consequently it was political dynamite. Manuel Vincente, CEO of Sonangol, who reported directly to the Head of State was very aware of this. Fernando Fonseca, his representative, was our direct contact person and participated in the weekly co-owners' monitoring meetings that I chaired. He went on to be appointed Minister of Town Planning.

This project turned out to be one of the most bizarre I had ever been involved in. I will not dwell on the various incidents, the numerous setbacks, the real estate developer's blows below the belt, his almost weekly claims, the arrogance of the general construction company and its misinterpretation of the specifications, or the conflicts between the architect and the developer concerning unpaid bills which culminated in the architect going on strike. Nor will I go into detail about Sonangol's ambiguous position, an unholy combination of construction company and co-owner, which allowed them to blow hot and cold during conflicts and occasionally torpedo the interests of the other two co-owners.

Suffice to say that we found ourselves in a permanent and exhausting state of conflict that we tried to manage with the limited means at our disposal. All this led to significant delivery delays. The project was finally completed two years after the deadline. The complex was inaugurated in person by President Santos in December 2009, two months after my departure.

All these problems were compounded by doubtless cases of corruption I got wind of. But as my friend Hanny, whom I met twice in Luanda where he did business and dealt with the same authorities, said: "Corruption? No, there is no corruption, we are simply told who to work with". Ever pragmatic, our legal adviser used the formula: "We have been directed".

It was crucial to make sure that my heavy responsibilities did not deliver me straight back into the talons of Demon Stress. Aware of this danger, I made an effort to share problems with my partners and superiors instead of keeping all my worries to myself.

In a way the project's complexity aided me in this: the construction team had about twenty people and as tasks were shared between several individuals it was easier to communicate and share. The project's political aspect also attracted a lot of interest from our management, both in Luanda and Houston. This was a very different situation from Chad and Cameroon where I had been more or less left to my own devices. Here, communication was practically daily and at all levels. Finally, I had an excellent partner in my Angolan colleague Amilton, a champion in communication and well aware of the local situation. I felt well supervised and supported in my tasks. All this helped me to manage the situation. Being able to share and quickly unload problems allowed me to put them into perspective. I learned from my past mistakes and the demon stayed in his box, well under control.

Physically, my condition continued to improve, albeit very slowly. I did the exercises recommended by the Splash physiotherapist in Amsterdam but probably not as much as I should have, as self-discipline was not always my forte. That's why I became a member of the gym at the Tropico hotel, which cost $ 1400 per year! At first I went there twice a week on average, but started to go less often. I mainly practiced weight-bearing exercises for my legs but when my subscription ran out, I did not renew it.

Occasionally, I took the stairs of my building – I was on the 7th floor – rather than the elevator. After a while, I tried running in my apartment which was spacious enough to allow this.

Every other Saturday I participated in "Hashes", group treks through the suburbs of Luanda. As well as giving me some physical exercise these outings were an excellent remedy against stress.[8]

The walks were confined to Luanda and its suburbs as the areas beyond this had not yet been cleared of mines. The long civil war had ended just six years earlier and much of the country was still covered in landmines. Thanks to these expeditions I was able to discover areas that I could never have ventured into alone. We often went through slums, where the poverty and dirt were in stark contrast to the wealth and cleanliness of the city centre. I took pictures on my phone and recorded them in a blog.[9]

Sometimes I felt down in the dumps when confronted with my disability: on inspection rounds of completed office areas I struggled to put on my plastic overshoes while standing, it was difficult to take big strides on certain construction sites visits or Hash hikes and my hands still trembled when I was nervous.

But by and large I remained optimistic, always convinced that in the long run I would make a full recovery and banish the demon.

I had come a long way. After all, I could easily have died if the wrong decisions had been taken in Lagos when the first symptoms appeared. I felt privileged to have this opportunity to start a new life.

LIBIDO

It was during this period of "new life" that I felt my libido return. At night, in my hotel room, I would commit the sin of Onan.

"The thingy apparently still works, which is a pleasant surprise. All the same weird, it feels weird. I can come but I don't ejaculate. I will need to discuss this with the doctor. After all, this was one of the very first symptoms of my illness." (Chad journal)

SEVILLE, SEPTEMBER 2009

I celebrated my 60th birthday in Spain with Wanda. We met in Seville, she flew from Amsterdam and I came from Luanda, where I was still working. Seville has a special meaning for me as my parents celebrated their honeymoon there in 1935. But this was my first visit to the city.

We spent our last night at the Hacienda de Benazuza, in San Lucas la Mayor, just outside Seville. It was a magical place. Formerly a farm, it had been transformed into a luxury hotel, with a one-storey building, several outbuildings, a Moorish-style building with arched porticos, shaded gardens with winding pathways, a refreshing swimming pool and large rooms decorated with period furniture. And, as a bonus, its restaurant was owned by the famous Catalan chef, Ferran Adria, renowned for his "molecular" cuisine. One of the delights we tasted was the famous soft olive that melts in your mouth. We laughed when I made a blunder, biting down on a razor shell, which I had mistaken for a biscuit. The impassive waiter, noting my error, swiftly replaced my plate without a word. This incident did not spoil the meal, which was simply magnificent.

All in all, it was a terribly romantic stay after which Wanda exclaimed: "I declare you are officially cured!"

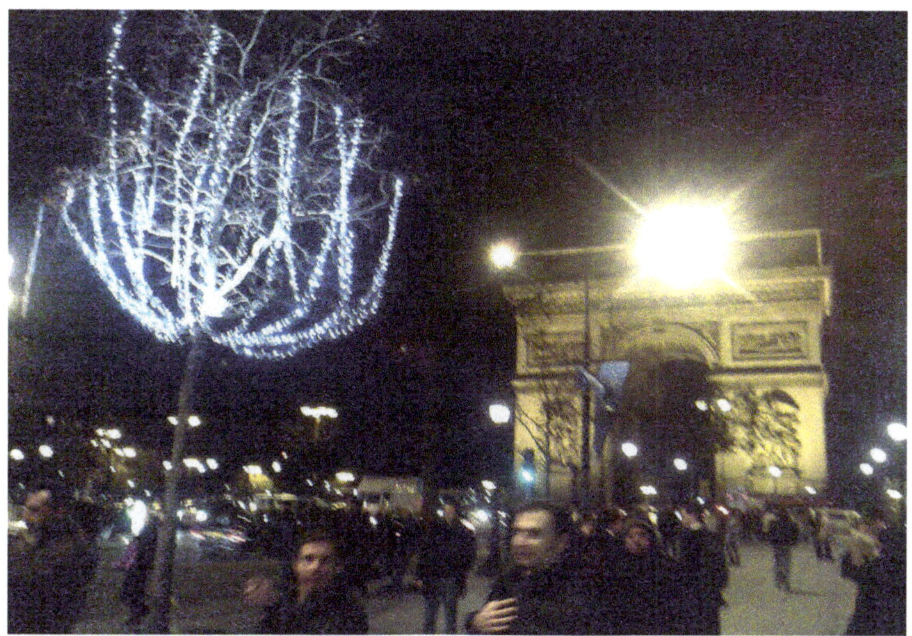

Paris, Champs Elysées, December 2007

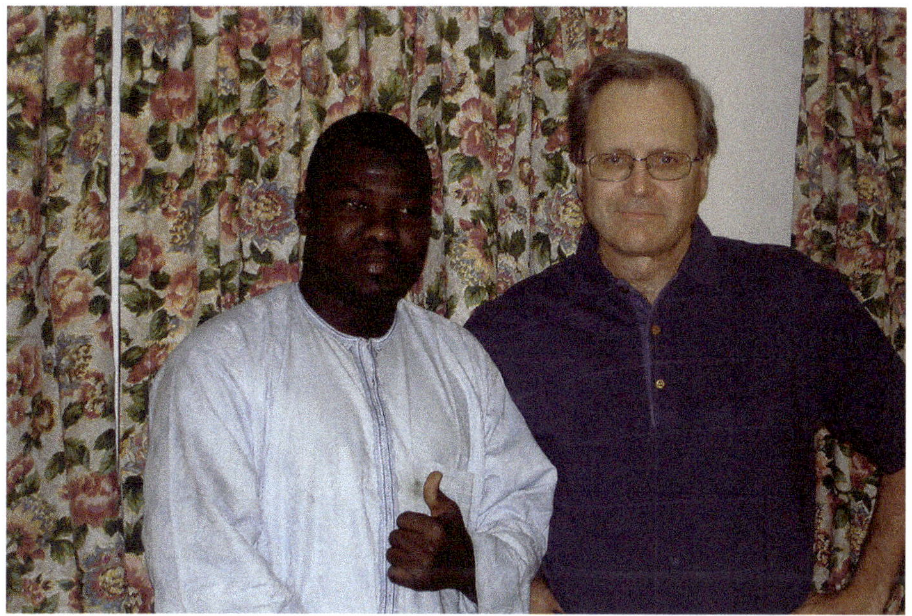

N'Djamena, with Mr Mohamed

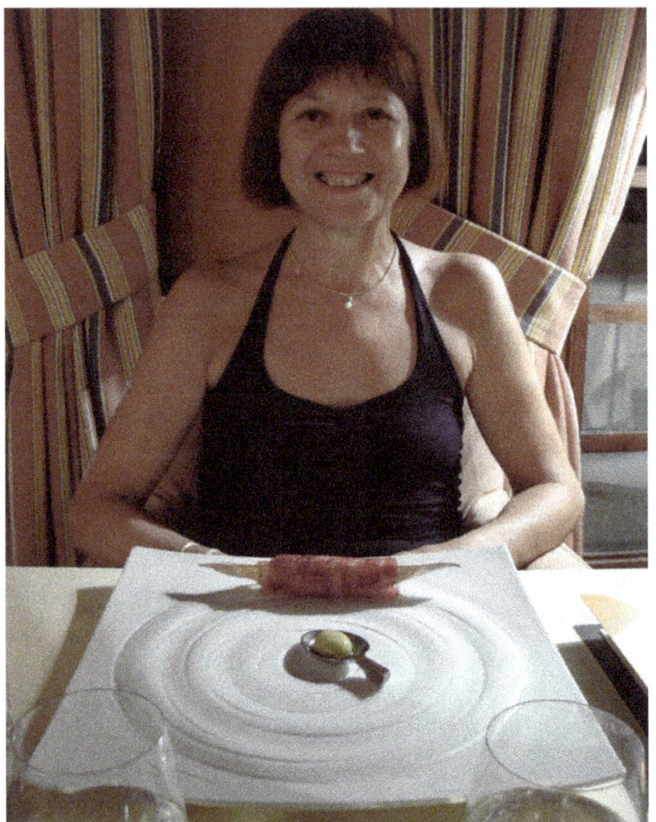

Wanda and the soft olive, Sevilla

CHAPTER SIX

TWELVE YEARS LATER

You need to tame this handicap, this alien which has entered us
– Michel Barras, paraplegic patient in 24 Hours of 09.05.2017

More than twelve years have elapsed since my "accident". Many things have happened during this period. After 18 months in Angola I was transferred in early 2010 first to Brisbane, Australia, then to Port Moresby, Papua New Guinea, for a new construction project. This time Wanda accompanied me and we spent five years of our life in this region of the world. We took advantage of this opportunity to discover countries that I had never thought I would see. In Australia we used to go on outings in Queensland every weekend and we spent my days off visiting the rest of the country. We also led a busy social life, organizing numerous barbecues with friends, acquaintances and colleagues from work. I spent the last two years in Port Moresby. Wanda stayed in Brisbane but joined me regularly in Papua so that we could explore this fascinating country together. All these activities enabled me to take some distance and put my professional life into perspective. As in Angola, I drew lessons from the past and was determined not to succumb to the sirens of stress.

Physically, I continued to make progress during this period, although it was not gigantic and could not be measured from one day to the next. I used landmarks to record it, such as the stairs of our house in Amsterdam or the climb towards Lina's in Le Trétien, places that we returned to during our annual visits to Europe. I could see some progress each time, but it was minimal.

When I returned to Europe four years ago, I resumed the physical training I had neglected in Australia. I did leg presses to strengthen my muscles and when we went to the mountains, I chose particularly steep areas for my walks. There were some real landmarks, such as the descent into the Trient Valley or the climb to the Emaney mountain pasture.

Today, 12 years later, I still have not recovered completely. My legs are weak and I can't climb steps higher than 25 centimetres without using my arms. Occasionally I have slight hand tremors when I make certain movements. When asked how I am doing I always say that I am well, that I am 90% recovered.

Since a couple of years I have not really noticed any significant progress. But I have not got any worse either. Have I reached the point of "no more progress" mentioned by the neurologist in Amsterdam 12 years ago?

I am however convinced I still can make some progress, even if minimal, and I am decided to keep on fighting, doing my exercises and being positive.

Anyway, I am beginning to realize that I will never recover totally, at least not in this life. Progress has practically ground to a halt. I will never be able to totally banish the demon. I will have to come to terms with it and live with it.

Somewhere inside me, a voice insists that I must tame this alien which has entered me.

EPILOGUE

The demon hasn't been totally banished, he is still here, albeit in a severely diminished form. I have learnt to co-exist with him. He lives in a small cage in a corner of the house, but the door is not padlocked. He is free to leave whenever he likes, but thankfully he does not appear often. I must say that I treat him gently: I do not indulge in excesses, I don't try to push myself past my limits, I rest after exertion and do my best to avoid stress. The demon seems to be satisfied by this, he appreciates being left in peace. We understand each other: in fact, you could almost say that we are on friendly terms. I have learned to accept him and live with him and I have him under control.

I have accepted that I will never recover entirely. But a 90% recovery is not bad at all. I have come a long way and would be in a much worse state now if my disease had not been diagnosed so quickly. I am terribly indebted to my doctors in Nigeria.

There are also plenty of positive aspects to this disease. It gave me the opportunity to spend time with my father during the last year of his life and it taught me that I needed to pay more attention to my friends and family. It also taught me to put work into perspective and to understand and overcome stress. Another unexpected bonus was that it led me to rediscover my country.

Mentally I am fine and I might say I fully accept my condition. To repeat what Ed Penniman, a colleague of misfortune, said: "I am 100% of what I can be". [10] I'm living a new life and I feel enriched by all the experiences this disease has brought me.

I saw Christiane Wilke recently. She's doing well, although she is not doing as well as I am. Her feet are still in splints, but she manages to move, using crutches if necessary. Her thumbs don't work well either.

She still has regular check-ups with Doctor Bogousslavski, because of insurance requirements, and they meet every six months. Christiane: "He is always happy with my modest progress and to this day he has never seen such a severe case. He repeats it every time".

Despite all this she has a positive attitude. She edits video films made during her many trips with her husband. They travel a lot, have recently completed a three-month cruise around the world, and they are now planning their next trip: the Trans-Siberian Express !

THE END

Amsterdam, December 2017/February 2019

POST SCRIPTUM

By sheer coincidence, I recently watched Ngos'a Bedimo (2013, 21 minutes), a short film by the Belgium-based artist Steven Jouwersma, It documents an attempt to form Cameroon's first heavy metal band in Douala, with an earnestness tinged with humour. Jouwersma, himself a musician, is the founder of this group.

The group is called Ngos'a Bedimo, meaning music of the ghosts. The band sings about traditional beliefs and local superstitions linked to witchcraft and occult practices.

At first sight heavy metal, dark and gloomy music born in the cold, grey, wet suburbs of Western Europe would seem to have little in common with the usually cheerful and festive character of Cameroonians, who are blessed with a warm and often sunny climate.

But Jouwersma explains that some Cameroonians associate this music with the summit of Mount Cameroon: a cold, dark, often rainy and misty region. To some, it is also a mystical place, said to be home to a colony of ghosts.

To find out more, Jouwersma climbed Mount Cameroon in two days. Once at the top, the guide refused to engage in the ritual to contact the spirits because Jouwersma had not brought the requisite bottle of whisky. Chilled to the bone by the bitter cold, they went back down again.

A few days later, on the night of their first performance at the nightclub "Mélodies d'Atant", the only member of the band to turn up was Dionkugu, the drummer. The other three members of the group were nowhere to be found. Jouwersma and Dionkugu decided to go it alone and they kicked up a hell of a din: they said that some passers-by outside the club thought there were at least twelve musicians inside.

The next day Jouwersma woke up with an eye infection and had to spend two days in hospital. The doctor told him that this was probably related to his ascent of Mount Cameroon.

Jouwersma never saw any of the other group members again: they had literally vanished into thin air. He suspected that they may have been put off by concerns about the taboos surrounding their music (some say that the group's name does not mean music of the ghosts but rather music of the devil). The spirit of the mountain and fear it inspired was too much for Ngos'a Bedimo.

I was particularly interested by the reference to Mount Cameroon in this anecdote. After all, wasn't it there that I had eaten the undercooked chicken that had probably led to my illness? I had not known that, according to superstition, the mountain was inhabited by ghosts. Were they the cause of my illness? Were there evil spirits or demons among them? Should I revise my story and include this new perspective?

Maybe the answer is to climb this mountain again in the hope of delivering myself permanently from the demon, returning it to its own world. Why not? But to do such a climb, I would first need to recover my strength, especially in my legs. This has not happened yet and maybe it never will. I am therefore faced with a dilemma: should I heal completely in order to climb or must I make the climb in order to heal completely? It's a diabolical dilemma. Is this not proof that the demon exists? At any rate, just in case, I will bring along a bottle of whisky.

NOTES

1. Fictitious name (forgot the real one)

2. Festival Onze Plus : Serge Wintsch and his wife Francine managed this festival until 2015. It has since then successfully been taken over by a new enthusiastic team.

3. To learn more about the Bogousslavsky case:

- Bibliopathe malgré lui, Edouard Launet, Libération 13 février 2010. Link: <http://www.liberation.fr/societe/2010/02/13/bibliopathe-malgre-lui_609698> - in French. A detailed report of the 2010 court case
- Voleurs par amour de l'art, Gilles Gaetner, Valeurs Actuelles, 29 avril 2010. Link: <www.valeursactuelles.com > accueil >> société >> voleurs par amour de l'art –
in French. A good summary of the case
- Numerous other reviews on Internet in both French and English can be consulted by simply googling on either "Lucien Bogousslavsky" ou "Serge Bogousslavsky"
- " L'Indifférent " by Jean-Antoine Watteau (1684-1721)

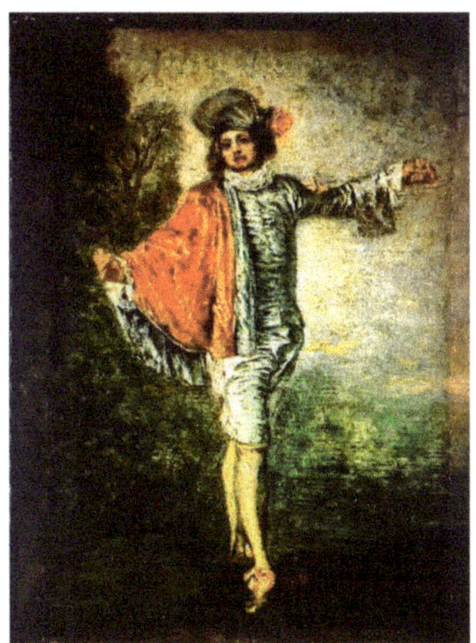

"L'Indifférent", 25x19 cm, c.1717, Musée du Louvre

The painting is also known as The Casual Lover. Shining folds of silk give the figure of carefree young man a delightful shimmer appropriate to his pose. He is about to execute a dance step. Watteau was always drawn to the inaugural moment of an action. The surface of this small panel suffered from clumsy restoration (source: Internet)

4. Maurice Béjart died 6 months later in Lausanne in December 2007 – he had heart and kidney problems but the cause of his passing was never disclosed.

5. The RCA denomination was amended in 2010 following a merger. Current denomination is Reade: centrum voor revalidatie geneeskunde en reumatologie in Amsterdam en omstreken.

6. Gallery WM (Wanda Michalak): Gallery run by my wife Wanda who is a photographer, located in Amsterdam. Website: <www.gallerywm.com>

7. Angola had just barely emerged from a brutal 27-year civil war that formally ended in 2002

8. The Hash House Harriers (HHH or H3) is an international group of non-competitive running social clubs. An event organised by a club is known as hash, hash run or simply hashing, with participants calling themselves hashers or hares and hounds (wikipedia). The Luanda section organised running as well as walking events.

9. Blog : Next Stop Papua New Guinea link : <https://paulcs.wordpress.com>

10. Ed Penniman was stricken at age 42 with Guillain-Barré Syndrome, which left him quadriplegic. In the years since he has recovered physically (still disabled but no longer a quadriplegic), psychologically and spiritually to become a new and more functional person than before the trauma. He published the book "You are up to you - Innovate a new self for a new life" (2016) relating his experience. A highly recommended book, available on Amazon. See also <www.youareuptoyou.com>.

ACKNOWLEDGMENTS

A big thanks to the following people for all their good advice, support and assistance:

Marie-Noëlle Mauris, Sabine Haximeri, Jean-François Jaton

Sebastian Rypson, Scott McCall, Pete Purnell

Harrie Blommesteijn, Raoul Balai, Leszek Sczaniecki

English translation: Armelle Desmarchelier

I also want to thank all family, friends and work colleagues for all their support and understanding, including those not specifically mentioned in the story.

A big thanks for all medics, therapists, paramedics, etc. who helped and assisted in the different phases of my recovery. These people are all heroes.

A special thanks to Christiane Wilke and Ed Penniman

And last but not least, a huge thanks to my wife Wanda for all her patience and on-going encouragement: "Come on, it's OK now: you are not ill anymore"